FUTURESCAN

Health Care Trends and Implications

2019–2024

T0206838

Leading Through Times of Change

by Ian Morrison, Ph.D.

As the nation's medical system goes through a period of high uncertainty and disruption, *Futurescan 2019–2024* brings together insightful experts and thought leaders to prepare hospitals and health systems for key trends that are shaping the future of health care.

Drug Crisis

Michael Botticelli, director of the White House Office of National Drug Control Policy under the Obama administration, is currently executive director of the Grayken Center for Addiction at Boston Medical Center.

In his article, Botticelli writes that "the nation's opioid epidemic is one of the defining crises of our time and requires a forceful response from every sector. For hospitals and health systems, the epidemic forces an even stronger sense of urgency given the magnitude of the problem and its intersection with hospital services." He says some hospitals are successfully responding to the challenge through efforts such as the following:

- Embracing nonopioid pain management practices.
- Enhancing the identification and treatment of patients with substance use disorders (SUDs).
- Incorporating SUD issues into payment and service delivery reform efforts.

Botticelli notes that "addressing the opioid crisis in the United States

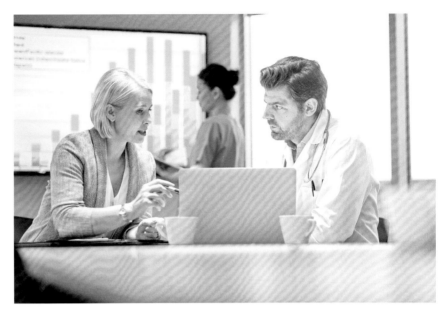

must be part of larger health care reform strategies, particularly those focused on containing costs, improving medical outcomes, enhancing population health and addressing social determinants of health."

Digital Health

Health care futurists Matthew Holt and Indu Subaiya, M.D., focus on emerging trends in digital health. Holt is the founder and publisher of *The Health Care Blog*, cofounder of the Health 2.0 conference and a founding principal of Health 2.0 Advisors. Subaiya is currently executive vice president of Health 2.0 and co-founder of Health 2.0: User Generated Healthcare.

They write, "The easy availability of cloud- and mobile-based computing systems has revolutionized the business sector, putting power and access into the hands of employees and customers and creating huge shifts in how transactions are done." Holt and Subaiya observe that health care organizations were "latecomers to the enterprise technology game" and are now playing catch-up. As technological advances accelerate, they urge leaders to be prepared for the next wave of change and its applications to hospitals and health systems, including blockchain, artificial intelligence (AI), virtual reality and augmented reality.

Their article also takes us through the likely focus of technology giants such as Amazon, Apple and Alphabet/Google as they grow their presence and impact in the field. Traditionally, the U.S. medical system has centered around care

About the Author

Ian Morrison, Ph.D., is an author, consultant and futurist. He received an undergraduate degree from the University of Edinburgh, Scotland; a graduate degree from the University of Newcastle upon Tyne, England; and an interdisciplinary doctorate in urban studies from the University of British Columbia, Canada. He is the author of several books, including the best-selling *The Second Curve: Managing the Velocity of Change*. Morrison is the former president of the Institute for the Future and a founding partner of Strategic Health Perspectives, a forecasting service for clients in the health care industry.

delivery, services and technology platforms, in that order. The authors invite us to "imagine inverting this triple-layer stack and starting with technology platforms." In this scenario, trackers and AI systems would monitor and even suggest next steps to clinicians and patients to improve the quality of care.

Holt and Subaiya stress that it is vital for health care leaders to understand these technologies and trends through learning and pilots and by engaging with clinical leaders in their organizations.

Biotechnology

Chad Bouton is director of the Center for Bioelectronic Medicine at the Feinstein Institute for Medical Research at Northwell Health and a renowned researcher and developer of advanced biomedical technology. Bouton explains in his article how this exciting new field combines neuroscience, molecular biology and bioengineering to tap into the nervous system to treat conditions involving inflammation, such as Crohn's disease, lupus, rheumatoid arthritis and paralysis.

He observes that while many of the advances in bioelectronic medicine are related to implantable devices, innovations in wearable technology will also play a major role in creating new therapies and treatments. And he says discoveries made in the lab are being made possible by investors from industry who recognize bioelectronics as a growing sector that will present alternatives to the biochemical therapies traditionally offered by Big Pharma to treat many diseases and conditions.

In the future, Bouton believes this branch of technology will continue to expand, and we can expect rapid growth in the field that could greatly improve how we deliver care.

Value-Based Care

As part of their America's Most Valuable Care study, David S. P. Hopkins, Ph.D., Melora Simon, Thomas Wang, Ph.D., and Arnold Milstein, M.D., of the Clinical Excellence Research Center at Stanford University have concentrated

on identifying hospitals that consistently provide high-value care—excellent quality at a low cost.

Their article highlights the results of the research, which revealed three sets of care delivery attributes that distinguish top-performing hospitals from their peers: (1) thinking beyond the hospital stay, (2) cutting waste, not safety and (3) engaging the frontline team in improving the cost-effectiveness of needed care.

The study found that hospitals are rapidly adopting these attributes in areas where they have the greatest economic incentive, such as readmissions and episodes of care. Stronger payer incentives will likely be necessary to increase adoption of attributes that reduce hospital occupancy.

The articles by this year's panel of experts provide evidence-based insights designed to help hospitals and health systems prepare for a range of strategic, market, policy, social, economic and competitive challenges.

The authors conclude, "As payers gradually increase rewards for yearlong excellence in care delivery, hospital and health system leaders will benefit from implementing best practices and bright spots in value-driven performance that meet the needs of patients and health insurers alike."

Physician Aggregation

Amir Dan Rubin, president and CEO of One Medical, begins his article on building physician networks through partnerships by emphasizing the rapid pace at which health care organizations are aligning with physicians.

He points out that in the latest *Futurescan* national survey of hospital and health system leaders, 76 percent of respondents say they are already growing their networks by more than 25 percent or are likely to do so in the next five years. He says the survey also indicates

that three-quarters of respondents are operating their network at a loss or are willing to do so to achieve broader strategic objectives.

According to Rubin, health systems are pursuing these investments to attract more covered lives to their networks; to deliver higher levels of service, access and value; and to prevent physicians and their patient bases from becoming aligned with competing networks.

One of the best ways to accomplish these goals, he says, is through partnerships, including affiliations, joint ventures, clinically integrated networks, lease arrangements, management services offerings, cost-plus contracts, fee-for-service billing and capitated or accountable care organization–like arrangements.

Many providers, he adds, find that these options can reduce capital burdens and business risks because all partnering organizations commit resources and management energy to the initiatives.

Governance

James E. Orlikoff, president of Orlikoff & Associates Inc. and a renowned expert on governance and the emerging health care environment, begins his article by stating that the traditional governance model "can no longer be taken for granted" in "the rapidly changing and radically challenging health care landscape."

He says hospital and health system boards are getting older: Since 2005, the percentage of board members under the age of 50 has declined. Furthermore, time demands on board members are growing and are an increasing cause of complaint.

Looking ahead, Orlikoff predicts leaders can expect the following:

- Recruiting and retaining qualified board members will become more difficult.
- Effectively integrating members of the millennial generation and Generation X into current governance models will be a growing problem.
- Leaders will experiment with new approaches to governance, with mixed results.

As the traditional model of governance nears the end of its useful life, Orlikoff says, "We must begin to conceptualize and then to experiment with new models that are relevant to a radically different future."

Policy and Regulation

Erin C. Fuse Brown, J.D., an associate professor of law and a faculty member of the Center for Law, Health and Society at the Georgia State University College of Law, provides an insightful perspective on the growing importance of the states' role in establishing health care policies and regulations.

Fuse Brown says that nearly a decade after the passage of the Affordable Care Act, political gridlock has made it difficult for the federal government to move forward with national reforms, while a renewed emphasis on state flexibility means states are stepping into the vacuum to take action on a variety of health care concerns.

She notes that the stakes are high because rising medical expenses translate to increasing budgetary pressure for states, squeezing out other public priorities such as education and infrastructure. In response, states are focusing on three key issues:

1. Rising costs from consolidation.
2. Drug price increases.
3. Affordability for health care consumers.

Fuse Brown concludes that the growing role of states will mean more state-by-state variation. Hospitals and health systems will need to concentrate not just on health care policies at the federal level but also on a proliferation of state regulations that will affect their facilities, finances and delivery models.

Workforce

Susan Salka, president and CEO of AMN Healthcare, leads the country's largest health care staffing and recruitment company. In her article, Salka describes the industry's unprecedented workforce shortages across the country as one of the most critical issues facing hospitals and health systems now and in the future.

She points out that the growing deficit of qualified physicians, nurses and many other medical professionals is driving problems related to hiring, retention, turnover, unit staffing and scheduling, morale, quality of care and overtime costs. According to Salka, health care employment continues to boom but still cannot keep pace with demand because of two leading drivers:

- An aging population that is consuming more health care services.
- The wave of retirements among baby boomer practitioners.

To help resolve the crisis, she calls for investment in modernizing the field's human resources sector. Salka says providers that use innovative best practices in recruitment and retention, coupled with hiring outside health care staffing experts when needed, is a formula for success in the escalating race for clinical talent.

Conclusion

Futurescan once again identifies key issues and emerging trends that demand an informed and planned response by health care leaders. The articles by this year's panel of experts provide evidence-based insights designed to help hospitals and health systems prepare for a range of strategic, market, policy, social, economic and competitive challenges and to guide them in taking the actions required to be successful in the ever-changing health care landscape.

Agents of Change: How Hospitals and Health Systems Can Change the Course of the Opioid Epidemic

by Michael Botticelli

The nation's opioid epidemic is one of the defining crises of our time and requires a forceful response from every sector. For hospitals and health systems, the epidemic forces an even stronger sense of urgency given the magnitude of the problem and its intersection with hospital services. Our ability to address the crisis depends to a large degree on how well the health care field implements evidence-based services, continues to innovate and replicates emerging best practices.

The stakes could not be higher. The number of drug overdose deaths involving opioids has risen sharply since the turn of the century, reaching more than 49,000 in 2017 (exhibit 1). The increase in overdose deaths is a major contributor to the shocking decline in life expectancy in the United States over the past two years (Xu et al. 2018).

In 2016, an estimated 2.1 million people aged 12 years or older met diagnostic criteria for an opioid use disorder (OUD) (SAMHSA 2017). This statistic may be a dramatic underestimation because overall prevalence is derived

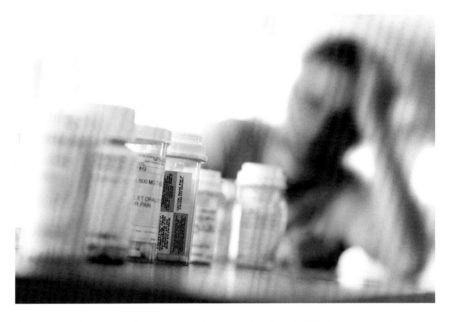

from national survey information and does not include homeless individuals or those who are currently incarcerated—populations known to have high OUD rates.

In addition, needle sharing and the lack of access to sterile syringes associated with heroin and fentanyl use have led to a dramatic increase in hepatitis C virus infections, as well as localized

outbreaks of HIV. In just over five years, the number of new hepatitis C infections reported to the Centers for Disease Control and Prevention (CDC) has nearly tripled, reaching a 15-year high (CDC 2018).

Another consequence has been a marked increase in the number of pregnant women with an OUD. From 2004 to 2014, the number of U.S. infants

About the Author

Michael Botticelli, one of the nation's leading addiction experts, is executive director of the Grayken Center for Addiction at Boston Medical Center. Previously, he was director of national drug control policy for the Obama administration. He joined the White House Office of National Drug Control Policy (ONDCP) as deputy director in November 2012 and later served as acting director. Botticelli has more than two decades of experience supporting Americans affected by substance use disorders.

Before joining ONDCP, he served as director of the Bureau of Substance Abuse Services at the Massachusetts Department of Public Health, where he expanded innovative and nationally recognized prevention, intervention, treatment and recovery services for Massachusetts. Botticelli holds a bachelor of arts degree from Siena College and a master of education degree from St. Lawrence University. He is also in long-term recovery from a substance use disorder, celebrating more than 28 years of recovery.

FUTURESCAN SURVEY RESULTS
Drug Crisis

How likely is it that the following will happen by 2024?

Already Happening (%)	Very Likely (%)	Somewhat Likely (%)	Neutral (%)	Somewhat Unlikely (%)	Very Unlikely (%)
30	28	24	12	4	3

Our organization will emphasize nonpharmacological pain management (e.g., acupuncture or cognitive behavioral therapy) to reduce opioid prescribing (e.g., number of prescriptions, duration or dosage) by physicians in our employment.

| 27 | 43 | 20 | 6 | 3 | 1 |

Our organization will expand the ability to diagnose patients who may have a substance use disorder while integrating treatment into multiple health care settings.

| 18 | 28 | 25 | 18 | 6 | 5 |

Our organization will integrate peers/recovery coaches into substance abuse and treatment services or other services such as emergency departments.

| 13 | 24 | 28 | 21 | 8 | 6 |

Expansion of accountable care organizations will serve as a major driver for an enhanced focus on substance use disorders among patient populations for our organization.

| 16 | 30 | 28 | 17 | 6 | 3 |

Our organization will establish initiatives specifically to meet the needs of employees or their family members addicted to opioids or other drugs.

Note: Percentages in each row may not sum exactly to 100 percent because of rounding.

What Health Care Executives Anticipate by 2024

- To decrease opioid prescribing by employed physicians, 58 percent of hospital and health system leaders either already are emphasizing nonpharmacological pain management alternatives or are very likely to do so.

- About two-thirds (65 percent) of respondents are at least somewhat confident that expansion of accountable care organizations will play a key role in enhancing the focus on patient substance use disorders.

- Sixteen percent of leaders have established their own organizational initiatives to help employees or their family members addicted to opioids or other drugs. Another 58 percent are somewhat or very likely to do so.

Exhibit 1

Number of Deaths Involving Opioids

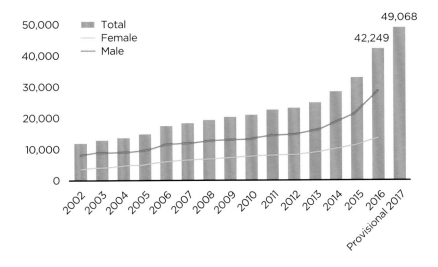

Source: National Institute on Drug Abuse (2018).

—*continued from pg. 5*

diagnosed with opioid withdrawal symptoms, known as neonatal abstinence syndrome, increased 433 percent—from 1.5 to 8.0 per 1,000 hospital births (Patrick et al. 2015).

The emergence of inexpensive, highly potent synthetic drugs, such as fentanyl and its analogues, adds a heartbreaking level of severity to opioid overdoses. From 2014 to 2016, the percentage of overdose deaths attributable to fentanyl increased from less than 20 percent to almost 50 percent (CDC 2016).

The impact of the opioid crisis on the health care delivery system is staggering from both a volume and a cost perspective. Hospitalizations related to opioid misuse and dependence have increased dramatically, with the rate of hospital inpatient stays per 100,000 population nearly doubling between 2000 and 2012. During that same period, opioid-related emergency department (ED) visits increased by 99.4 percent (Weiss et al. 2017). Because untreated addiction is a major driver of overall medical expenditures, hospitals and health systems have significant opportunities to identify and engage people in treatment—not only to achieve better outcomes for patients but also to reduce the large-scale financial burden.

The economic impact on our nation is also profound. A report by the White House's Council of Economic Advisers (2017) has estimated that opioid use in the United States is associated with more than $500 billion a year

in health care and criminal justice expenses, not to mention lost business productivity—nearly 2.8 percent of the gross domestic product.

How We Got Here

The epidemic that now claims close to 140 lives a day grew out of a number of intersecting dynamics. It took decades to develop, with many historical factors combining to make conditions ripe for this epidemic to flourish:

- A fragmented health care delivery system.
- An overreliance on arrest and incarceration at both the policy and funding levels.
- A lack of training among medical staff on substance use disorders (SUDs).
- Inadequate reimbursement and insurance coverage for SUD treatment.
- The pervasive stigma surrounding drug users.

As a result of these and other factors, only a very small percentage of those with an SUD receive care.

Historically, the country's policies and funding for dealing with the problem and its consequences focused heavily on reducing global drug supply and on law enforcement at the federal, state and local levels. Until 2012, public health approaches such as prevention, early intervention and treatment were not high priorities.

In addition, one of the early drivers of the epidemic was the overprescribing of opioid medications. According to the CDC, doctors wrote 72.4 opioid prescriptions per 100 persons in 2006. This rate increased 4.1 percent annually from 2006 to 2008 and 1.1 percent annually from 2008 to 2012. By that year, 259 million opioid prescriptions were written in the United States—four times as many as in 1999. Although we have seen an overall decrease since 2012, the level of opioid prescribing still remains triple what it was in 1999 (Guy et al. 2017).

From the beginning, one of the primary obstacles in the path to stopping the opioid epidemic has been the fact that too few people with opioid addiction are receiving the help they need. According to the National Survey on Drug Use and Health, only 10 to 14 percent of those with an SUD receive treatment (SAMHSA 2017). Despite the high prevalence of people with SUDs intersecting with the nation's health care delivery system, only 8 percent of the referrals are coming from health care settings. One major cause of the low treatment rate is a lack of clinical education in medical curricula on the issue. A 2012 study on the gap between the science and the practice of addiction medicine found the topic hardly mentioned in the board certification exam requirements of several key medical specialties (Center on Addiction 2012).

This lack of training created significant missed opportunities to identify people with or at risk for SUDs. Similar to chronic diseases such as diabetes, drug addiction can be linked to family history, detected early and treated with evidence-based therapies. Yet, in the mid- to late 2000s, as opioid abuse increased, little detection or intervention occurred in hospitals and primary care settings.

In a national survey of primary care providers and psychiatrists, 18 percent of physicians reported that they typically offer no intervention to their alcoholic patients—not even a referral—in part because of misplaced concern about patients' sensitivity to these issues. Nearly the same proportion (15 percent)

reported that they do not intervene when use of illicit drugs is detected. Only 28.6 percent of family medicine residency programs have required addiction medicine curricula (Friedmann, McCullough and Saitz 2001).

Until the Affordable Care Act and Medicaid expansion in some states required an SUD treatment benefit, lack of insurance was a major barrier for many people seeking care. Compounding the problem, numerous public and commercial health plans had implemented a variety of discriminatory practices for SUD benefits that did not apply to other medical benefits. The 2008 Mental Health Parity and Addiction Equity Act attempted to rectify this inequity by requiring insurers to offer mental health and SUD benefits on a par with benefits for other medical conditions. Despite enhanced regulatory oversight and compliance efforts at both the state and federal levels, much work remains if we are to achieve full parity. Doing so will significantly increase the number of people who receive adequate treatment.

Insurance carve-out arrangements for SUDs can also present a significant barrier to identification and treatment because they segregate care delivery and payment despite evidence that many people with addictions have comorbid medical conditions and are high utilizers of medical services. The situation continues to drive episodic hospitalizations and other drains on the overall health care system. Yet, with separate payment streams, carve-out carriers have little incentive to promote ample treatment options for SUDs.

Changing History

The opioid crisis has reached a reckoning point. We must assess and rapidly replicate what evidence suggests is working. Ending the opioid epidemic will involve cumulative action on the part of multiple stakeholders, including the pharmaceutical industry, government, law enforcement sector and health care delivery system.

Given the burgeoning volume of inpatients and outpatients with an

OUD, hospitals have an opportunity to make a major impact on reducing morbidity and mortality related to the epidemic. The following examples illustrate how some hospitals are responding to the need.

Embracing nonopioid pain management practices. Nora Volkow, MD, director of the National Institute on Drug Abuse, has said that the overprescribing of opioids "started the fire." (Boston Medical Center 2018). It follows that, to extinguish the fire, we must continue to push for pain management strategies that rely on nonopioid medications and nonpharmacological approaches. These efforts go hand in hand with prescription-monitoring programs for problematic prescribing and reducing drug diversion. Some states have laws that limit doctors to prescribing a set course of opioids, but the hope is that the field will take action ahead of the mandates to adopt guidelines and standards that limit prescriptions and promote alternative pain management therapies.

After researchers at Dartmouth-Hitchcock in New Hampshire found that surgical patients need only 43 percent of the opioid pain medications they are generally prescribed, the hospital introduced new guidelines to reduce prescriptions and encourage over-the-counter alternatives. Results published in the journal *Annals of Surgery* reported a 53 percent reduction in the number of pills prescribed for five common outpatient procedures. Hospitals following this example must provide access to nonopioid medications and evidence-based, nonpharmacological pain management services (Hill et al. 2018).

Enhancing patient identification and treatment initiation. Beyond prescribing limits and vigilant monitoring, America's Essential Hospitals notes that hospitals are uniquely positioned to screen for and monitor opioid use by patients, offer transitional treatment and form multisector partnerships—all of which can have a significant impact on identifying and initiating treatment for patients with SUDs.

Approximately 15 percent of inpatients have an active SUD. Thus, hospitals have an opportunity to begin addiction treatment for those patients during their stay. Best-practice approaches include the Addiction Consult Service program at Boston Medical Center, which diagnoses and initiates care for patients with SUDs and links them to outpatient addiction treatment. This program has proven effective at the medical center in reducing subsequent hospitalizations and ED visits among that patient population (Trowbridge et al. 2017).

A recent Yale University study indicates that beginning treatment in EDs is another practice that should be more widely implemented in hospitals. The research found that patients with OUDs are more likely to receive addiction treatment and reduce opioid use long-term if they start medication to reduce cravings in the ED (D'Onofrio et al. 2015).

Despite the evidence, this practice is far from standard. Even though findings from a June 2018 study funded by the National Institute on Drug Abuse showed that opioid overdose deaths decreased by 59 percent for those receiving methadone and 38 percent for those receiving buprenorphine in the 12 months following a nonfatal overdose, fewer than one-third of patients were provided any medication for their OUD (Larochelle et al. 2018). Hospitals and health systems can help increase these percentages by encouraging more physicians to obtain Drug Enforcement Administration waivers to prescribe addiction medications. Currently, only 3 percent of primary care doctors have

gone through the necessary training, and even fewer actually prescribe.

Hospitals are also uniquely positioned to build their own treatment capacity in primary care settings. In Massachusetts, a primary care office–based opioid treatment program that

---

Ending the opioid epidemic will involve cumulative action on the part of multiple stakeholders, including the pharmaceutical industry, government, law enforcement sector and health care delivery system.

---

emphasizes collaborative care was created and is widely used across the nation through the Community Health Center Network.

Incorporating SUD issues into payment and service delivery reform efforts. Finally, addressing the opioid crisis in the United States must be part of larger health care reform strategies, particularly those focused on containing costs, improving medical outcomes, enhancing population health and addressing social determinants of health. Research shows that 20 percent of the factors leading to premature death are related to social and environmental issues, and 40 percent are related to behaviors (Committee on Population et al. 2015). Acknowledging this fact, hospitals and health systems are increasingly supporting community-based outreach programs and wellness initiatives.

For example, Rush University Medical Center in Chicago uses an online tool called NowPow to connect people who have chronic diseases with local resources that can help them better manage their conditions. According to *Modern Healthcare*, NowPow, which

grew out of a population health initiative led by the Lindau Lab at the University of Chicago, can also measure whether referrals were acted on and lets hospitals know how successful they were in assisting individuals with their needs (Dickson 2018).

Conclusion

From a historical perspective, the costs and casualties of today's opioid crisis might seem surreal to future generations. Hopefully, decades from now, this public health emergency will have been addressed through medical breakthroughs, health care innovations and provider- and community-based interventions. But for now, we remain far from this goal, and the severity of the problem warrants unprecedented action on the part of our hospitals, health systems and all those who are best positioned to reverse and eliminate the epidemic.

References

Boston Medical Center. 2018. "Boston University and the Grayken Center Host National Conversation on Research, Practice and the Opioid Epidemic." Accessed December 17. www.bmc.org/node?page=15.

Center on Addiction. 2012. "Addiction Medicine: Closing the Gap Between Science and Practice." Published June. www.centeronaddiction.org/addiction-research/reports/addiction-medicine-closing-gap-between-science-and-practice.

Centers for Disease Control and Prevention (CDC). 2018. "Surveillance for Viral Hepatitis—United States, 2016." Updated April 16. www.cdc.gov/hepatitis/statistics/2016surveillance/.

———. 2016. "Synthetic Opioid Overdose Data." Updated December 16. www.cdc.gov/drugoverdose/data/fentanyl.html.

Committee on Population, Division of Behavioral and Social Sciences and Education, Board on Health Care Services, National Research Council and Institute of Medicine. 2015. "Data from Major Studies of Premature Mortality." Published February 24. www.ncbi.nlm.nih.gov/books/NBK279981/.

Council of Economic Advisers. 2017. "The Underestimated Cost of the Opioid Crisis." Published November. www.whitehouse.gov/briefings-statements/cea-report-underestimated-cost-opioid-crisis/.

Dickson, V. 2018. "Mapping the Impact of Social Determinants of Health." *Modern Healthcare*. Published March 31. www.modernhealthcare.com/article/20180331/NEWS/180339986.

D'Onofrio, G., P.G. O'Connor, M.V. Pantalon, M.C. Chawarski, S.H. Busch, P.H. Owens, S.L. Bernstein and D.A. Fiellin. 2015. "Emergency Department–Initiated Buprenorphine/Naloxone Treatment for Opioid Dependence: A Randomized Clinical Trial." *Journal of the American Medical Association* 313 (16): 1636–44.

Friedmann, P.D., D. McCullough and R. Saitz. 2001. "Screening and Intervention for Illicit Drug Abuse: A National Survey of Primary Care Physicians and Psychiatrists." *Archives of Internal Medicine* 161 (2): 248–51.

Guy, J.G., K. Zhang, M.K. Bohm, J. Losby, B. Lewis, R. Young, L.B. Murphy and D. Dowell. 2017. "Vital Signs: Changes in Opioid Prescribing in the United States, 2006–2015." *Morbidity and Mortality Weekly Report* 66 (26): 697–704.

Hill, M.V., R.S. Stucke, M.L. McMahon, J.L. Beeman and R.J. Barth Jr. 2018. "An Educational Intervention Decreases Opioid Prescribing After General Surgical Operations." *Annals of Surgery* 267 (3): 468–72.

Larochelle, M.R., D. Bernson, T. Land, T.J. Stopka, N. Wang, Z. Xuan, S.M. Bagley, J.M. Leibschutz and A.Y. Walley. 2018. "Medication for Opioid Use Disorder After Nonfatal Opioid Overdose and Association with Mortality: A Cohort Study." *Annals of Internal Medicine* 169 (3): 137–45.

National Institute on Drug Abuse. 2018. "Overdose Death Rates." Revised August. www.drugabuse.gov/related-topics/trends-statistics/overdose-death-rates.

Patrick, S.W., M.M. Davis, C.U. Lehmann and W.O. Cooper. 2015. "Increasing Incidence and Geographic Distribution of Neonatal Abstinence Syndrome: United States, 2009 to 2012." *Journal of Perinatology* 35 (8): 650–55.

Substance Abuse and Mental Health Services Administration (SAMHSA). 2017. "Results from the 2016 National Survey on Drug Use and Health." Published September 7. www.samhsa.gov/data/sites/default/files/NSDUH-DetTabs-2016/NSDUH-DetTabs-2016.pdf.

Trowbridge, P., Z.M. Weinstein, T. Kerensky, P. Roy, D. Regan, J.H. Samet and A.Y. Walley. 2017. "Addiction Consultation Services—Linking Hospitalized Patients to Outpatient Addiction Treatment." *Journal of Substance Abuse Treatment* 79: 1–5.

Weiss, A.J., A. Elixhauser, M.L. Barrett, C.A. Steiner, M.K. Bailey and L. O'Malley. 2017. "Opioid-Related Inpatient Stays and Emergency Department Visits by State, 2009–2014." Healthcare Cost and Utilization Project. Revised January. www.hcup-us.ahrq.gov/reports/statbriefs/sb219-Opioid-Hospital-Stays-ED-Visits-by-State.jsp.

Xu, J., S.L. Murphy, K.D. Kochanek, B. Bastian and E. Arias. 2018. "Deaths: Final Data for 2016." *National Vital Statistics Reports* 67 (5): 1–75.

Flipping the Stack: Can New Technology Drive Health Care's Future?

by Matthew Holt and Indu Subaiya, M.D.

The easy availability of cloud- and mobile-based computing systems has revolutionized the business sector, putting power and access into the hands of employees and customers and creating huge shifts in how transactions are done. Now the companies with the highest market value are both the drivers *and* the beneficiaries of this transition—notably Apple, Facebook, Amazon and Alphabet (Google), as well as their international rivals such as Samsung, Baidu, Tencent and Alibaba.

Underpinning this transformation has been a change from enterprise-specific software to generic cloud-based services—sometimes called SMAC (social, mobile, analytics and cloud). Applications for data storage, sales management and email and the hardware they ran on were put into enterprises in the client-server era dominated by Intel and Microsoft. These have now migrated to cloud-based, on-demand services, and consumers and businesses alike

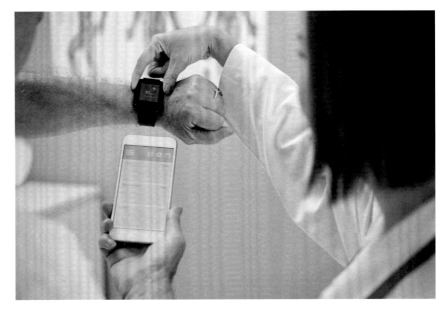

have flocked to these new platforms using GSuite, Amazon Web Services, Salesforce, Slack and countless others (exhibit 1). Those technologies, in turn, have enabled the growth of completely new types of businesses, transforming sectors such as transportation (Uber), entertainment (Netflix), lodging (Airbnb) and more.

What About Health Care Organizations?

Hospitals and health systems were latecomers to the enterprise technology

About the Authors

Matthew Holt is a nationally recognized health technology expert who is best known as the founder of *The Health Care Blog* and cofounder of the Health 2.0 conference. *The Health Care Blog* has been a leading source of opinion, news and interviews about health and health technology since 2003 and features Holt's "Health in 2 Point 00" videos with Jessica DaMassa. Health 2.0 is the leading conference series showcasing frontier technologies in health care. Holt also works on SMACK.health, advising a group of startups navigating the health care world. Earlier in his career, following graduate work at Stanford University, Holt worked for the renowned Institute for the Future and the Harris Insights & Analytics polling organization.

Indu Subaiya, M.D., is a visionary leader whose work builds community, creates dialogue and inspires radical thinking about how health shapes lives. She cofounded and served as CEO of Health 2.0, the leading conference and media platform that promotes and catalyzes new technologies in health care. Health 2.0's conference business was acquired by HIMSS in 2017, and Subaiya continues to head the organization as executive vice president as it scouts new technologies and builds initiatives to drive sustainable change in today's health care landscape. An immigrant from India, Subaiya is a passionate advocate for ending health care disparities and increasing diversity in the industry's leadership ranks.

Digital Health

How likely is it that the following will happen by 2024?

Already Happening (%)	Very Likely (%)	Somewhat Likely (%)	Neutral (%)	Somewhat Unlikely (%)	Very Unlikely (%)
8	29	24	25	3	1

Our organization will use the FHIR (Fast Healthcare Interoperability Resources) standard to make accessing health care records easier for third-party applications and organizations.

6	24	27	36	6	2

Our organization will change most data storage and transaction tools to blockchain or other distributed computing technologies.

9	38	26	11	13	3

A major technology company, such as Google, Amazon or Apple, will emerge as a significant developer of health care services that competes directly with our organization's services.

Note: Percentages in each row may not sum exactly to 100 percent because of rounding.

What Health Care Executives Anticipate by 2024

- Nearly half (47 percent) of hospital and health system leaders say a major technology company either already has emerged as a competitor to their organization's health care services or is very likely to do so.

- Fifty-seven percent of respondents are at least somewhat likely to change most of their organization's data storage and transaction tools to blockchain or other distributed computing technologies.

- Only 8 percent of leaders indicate that their organization uses the FHIR (Fast Healthcare Interoperability Resources) standard to facilitate access to health care records by third-party applications and organizations. However, another 53 percent say their organization is at least somewhat likely to do so.

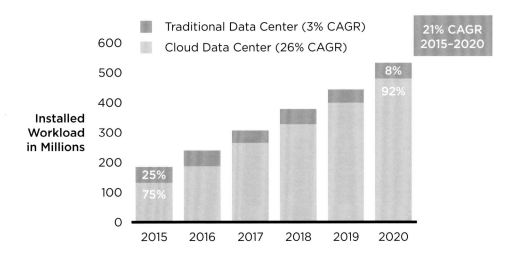

Exhibit 1

Growth in Use of Cloud Data Centers Versus Traditional Data Centers

Traditional Data Center (3% CAGR)
Cloud Data Center (26% CAGR)

21% CAGR
2015-2020

Installed Workload in Millions

600
500
400
300
200
100
0

25%
75%

8%
92%

2015 2016 2017 2018 2019 2020

Note: CAGR = compound annual growth rate.
Source: Cisco Global Cloud Index, 2015–2020.

—continued from pg. 11

game, including to client-servers. In the 2000s and 2010s, mostly in response to the HITECH (Health Information Technology for Economic and Clinical Health) Act, hospitals added electronic medical records (EMRs) to their other information systems. The majority of these EMRs are client-server based and enterprise specific. Even those that are cloud based tend to be hosted in the private cloud environment of vendors. However, the health care sector is likely to transition to using the cloud as other businesses have. Current technology vendors, including Epic and Cerner, are beginning to open their systems and are moving their clients to their private cloud, while another large vendor, Allscripts, has put most of its technology onto Microsoft's public cloud (Azure). Meanwhile, all of the major EMR vendors have adopted the FHIR (Fast Healthcare Interoperability Resources) standard and SMART (Substitutable Medical Apps and Reusable Technology)-on-FHIR protocols, which make it much easier to transfer data between different applications and to give users a choice of tools, many of which are hosted on the cloud.

How quickly is FHIR being adopted? In the *Futurescan* national survey, only 8 percent of health care executives said their organizations are already using FHIR to make it easier for third-party applications to access their data; 29 percent indicated they are very likely to do so by 2024,

and 24 percent reported they are somewhat likely. Our take is that these numbers understate FHIR's impact. After all, this standard is already being used by Apple to extract data for its health record from more than 100 top hospitals, and all major EMR vendors (and many major health systems) are developing a series of partnerships, app stores and innovation programs to allow those third-party application vendors easier access to users (e.g., clinicians, patients, administrators). Also, many hospitals are contributing to the explosion in apps and services by encouraging their internal teams to create them.

There is considerable debate among experts regarding the near-term evolution of technology in health care. Most hospitals have spent huge amounts on EMR installations in recent years, so they are unlikely to replace their incumbent vendors. But although the transaction layer inside the current EMR may seem to be well embedded in the system, new types of interface, storage and data analytics solutions are increasingly being trialed.

The advent of FHIR and distributed storage certainly portends a future of decentralized data and services, with big implications for hospitals and health systems that are trying to implement physical and contractual controls over those areas.

New Developments

As the pace of technological advances continues to accelerate, health care leaders need to be

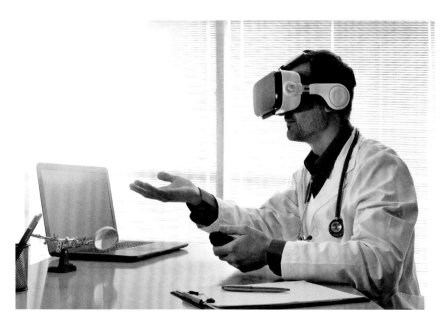

prepared for the next wave of change and how it will affect their organizations and the communities they serve.

At the forefront are blockchain, artificial intelligence (AI), virtual reality (VR) and augmented reality (AR)—all built on the expanding capabilities of cloud computing and driven by the burgeoning internet of things (IoT).

Blockchain. Blockchain is a distributed database technology in which every transaction is recorded on every node in a network. It is, therefore, hard to hack or alter. Blockchain also does more than just record transactions: It allows "smart contracts" to be embedded in the blockchain to enable permissions, grant access to data and perform transactions—all automatically. Closely related is the concept of "identity by consensus," which enables the authorization of identity from data gathered from multiple sources.

Blockchain is still in its early days. One or two industry groups are forming in health care, including the Linux Foundation's Hyperledger Consortium and Hashed Health. In a recent survey, 75 percent of health care executives described their understanding of blockchain as "excellent," while 39 percent indicated that learning about blockchain is one of their top five priorities. Eleven percent of respondents reported deploying blockchain somewhere in their enterprise (Deloitte 2018).

In the latest *Futurescan* survey, 6 percent of hospital and health system leaders said their organization has already changed most of its data storage and transaction tools to blockchain or other distributed computing technologies. Another 24 percent believe such a change is very likely in the next five years.

Artificial intelligence. The only thing generating more hype than blockchain is AI. At its core, AI enables very quick computation of vast amounts of data, looks for patterns and makes suggestions about them (e.g., symptom assessment in radiology) or, in some cases, acts on them (e.g., self-driving cars, fully robotic surgery). Perhaps the most promising area for AI in health care is in computations that are just far too complicated for humans, such as identifying the factors behind cancer or managing complex drug regimens for safety and matching them with genomes and phenotypes.

AI is also being used for tasks such as the following:

- Predicting which patients are likely to contract a certain disease based on lab, medical and insurance claims data.
- Personalizing drug regimens to lower patients' risk for complex interactions and to improve outcomes.
- Leveraging chatbot technology to analyze patient symptoms and diagnose health problems.

Virtual reality and augmented reality. While VR and AR are already changing the worlds of gaming and entertainment, it is more difficult to see where these technologies fit in health care. So far, VR is being experimented with in pain management and mental health. AR seems to be finding its niche in remotely recording and supporting patient–physician visits and overlaying X-ray images on patients to aid in clinical precision.

The AI, VR and AR revolution is likely to make its biggest impact when these trends are combined with the underlying technologies of sensors, analytics and on-demand computing. The early stages of this potential have been dominated by consumer use of voice assistants and automatically controlled systems that respond to questions and commands. Some companies are already putting voice assistants in hospital rooms to replace nurse call systems. Soon, more of these communications will be automated, and the sensors will not only take instruction but also passively track patient activity in the hospital or home and automatically respond.

The Role of the Tech Giants

It has escaped few observers' attention that the companies with the most advanced technology in AI, voice recognition, sensors and cloud computing are the same ones that have benefited from the SMAC revolution. The health tech press has been abuzz with articles attempting to read the tea leaves about what Apple, Amazon and Alphabet (Google) will do in the health care sector in the future (see sidebar).

The *Futurescan* survey asked executives whether they believe a major technology company will emerge as a significant developer of health care services that compete directly with hospitals and health systems. Only 9 percent of respondents said this is already happening (which might be a surprise to the tech giants), but another 38 percent indicated it is very likely to happen in the next five years.

Although it remains to be seen how the tech giants' health care strategies will unfold, clearly they have the talent, resources and funding to make a considerable impact in the field. In addition, other major players such as CVS/Aetna, Walmart and UnitedHealth Group, to name a few, are not sitting still. All of them seem to be angling in on chronically ill consumers in the home—a patient population and location that health care providers have traditionally struggled with.

Inverting the Stack

New market entrants can change health care in several obvious scenarios, but the one in which they take a major role is called "inverting the stack."

Traditionally, the U.S. health care system has been designed around care delivery, services and technology platforms, in that order (exhibit 2).

Imagine inverting this triple-layer stack and starting with technology platforms (exhibit 3). In this model, sensors, trackers and AI systems and processes would be in place monitoring, measuring and suggesting next steps to both providers and patients. Health care would shift from being an event-driven system to a consistent process. Normal patient behavior and activity would not need a response, whereas exceptions and problems would require medical intervention from a combination of human- and machine-driven services. Health care delivery as we know it today would

be the final step (or layer in the stack). In fact, almost any intervention could be considered a failure of the system, or at least a correction of the autopilot mode.

What might this inverted stack look like? Imagine a combination of home-delivered medications (PillPack), IoT sensors recording a person's vital signs (Apple), technology-based services monitoring chronically ill patients (Livongo), online physician care (Doctors on Demand) or even acute, hospital-like care provided in the home (Medically Home). In this model, the tech platform is the underlying system, with services and professionals at the top of the stack. In our opinion, this scenario could soon become a reality that radically reduces doctor visits and hospital admissions and improves patient care.

Implications for Health Care Leaders

As the technology trends described in this article progress, the key question is how quickly and to what extent they will transform health care. Here are a few suggestions to help hospital and health system executives better understand the transition and assess the rate of change:

- Become familiar with the technologies. You will not fully understand VR by

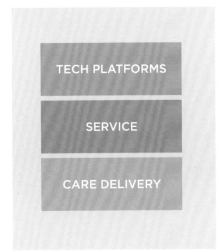

Exhibit 2

Traditional Health Care Model

TECH PLATFORMS

SERVICE

CARE DELIVERY

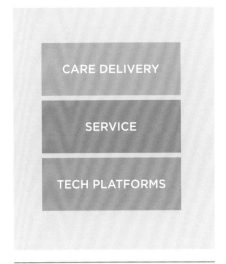

Exhibit 3

Tech Inverts the Stack

CARE DELIVERY

SERVICE

TECH PLATFORMS

reading about it. You might if you play a video game with your kids on their new Oculus headset.

- Talk to the clinicians who are using these new tools in your organization to get their feedback. Engage the end users—your patients—about their experiences in being treated with the technologies. Ask your researchers and analysts for data on the impact the technologies are having on the cost and quality of care.

- Spend time with health tech startups at conferences, participate in a health care incubator program and get to know the tech-savvy doctors in your hospital. They will be pushing the boundaries of technological innovation and know what may be possible in the future.
- Pay attention to both leading-edge payers (e.g., Oscar Health or any employer who uses Grand Rounds) and the Centers for Medicare & Medicaid Services. The more

payment-for-value becomes ingrained in health care, the likelier it is that real changes in how chronically ill patients are monitored and managed will be implemented.

Taking these steps is a good way to start preparing yourself for the next phase of health care's digital revolution and determining what strategies may or may not make sense for your organization now and in the future.

Reference

Deloitte. 2018. "2018 Global Blockchain Survey." Accessed September 20. www2.deloitte.com/us/en/pages/consulting/articles/innovation-blockchain-survey.html.

Bioelectronic Medicine: Creating New Treatment Paradigms

by Chad Bouton

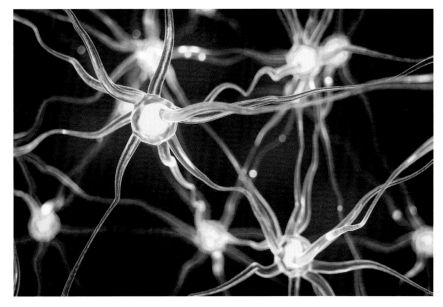

I n the new era of medicine, technology is woven into virtually every aspect of patient care. Electronic health records are being harnessed to identify ways to improve care, with predictive algorithms under development to warn providers about possible health issues. Advances in wearable devices help both patients and medical professionals track vital health information, while new laboratory instrumentation and artificial intelligence aid in applications ranging from detecting infections to diagnosing cancer.

A rapidly growing field called bioelectronic medicine uses technology to modulate the nervous system to treat disease and injury without the use of pharmaceuticals. Initial clinical trial results are positive and show the innovation is on its way to being a tangible alternative to certain medications. While it is hard to predict what will happen with this technology in the next few years, health care leaders should make it a priority to stay abreast of new developments because bioelectronics could radically alter how physicians, hospitals, health systems and other providers deliver care in the future.

Health care organizations that have a research component should also be aware of the field because research related to bioelectronic medicine has the potential to attract additional outside investment from donors and industry.

Harnessing the Nervous System to Treat Disease and Injury

Before delving into what the future holds, let's examine the foundation of bioelectronic medicine and some of its recent discoveries to understand how it differs from pharmaceutical research and development.

One of the initial discoveries was made in the late 1990s by Kevin J. Tracey, M.D., president and CEO of the Feinstein Institute for Medical Research, who found that the vagus nerve is involved in controlling inflammation (Tracey 2002). This revelation raised hope that if we can interact with the nervous system, we may be able to treat conditions involving inflammation, such as Crohn's disease, lupus and rheumatoid arthritis (RA). We may also be able to treat other conditions that involve

About the Author

Chad Bouton is the vice president of advanced engineering and director of the Center for Bioelectronic Medicine at the Feinstein Institute for Medical Research, the research arm of Northwell Health in New York. He formerly served as research leader at Battelle Memorial Institute, the world's largest independent research and development (R&D) organization, where he spent 18 years researching and developing biomedical technology. At the Feinstein Institute, Bouton is performing groundbreaking research in neurotechnology to treat paralysis and is developing new technologies to accelerate the field of bioelectronic medicine. His pioneering work, which allowed a paralyzed person to regain movement using a brain implant for the first time, has been featured on CBS's *60 Minutes*. Bouton holds more than 70 patents worldwide, and his technologies have received three R&D 100 Awards. Bouton was recognized by the U.S. Congress for his work in the medical device field, and Battelle has named him a Distinguished Inventor and an Inventor of the Year.

FUTURESCAN SURVEY RESULTS
Biotechnology

How likely is it that the following will happen by 2024?

Already Happening (%)	Very Likely (%)	Somewhat Likely (%)	Neutral (%)	Somewhat Unlikely (%)	Very Unlikely (%)
1	18	31	29	13	9

Our organization will use "smart clothing," both inside and outside the hospital, with embedded electronics for patient care, such as shirts that monitor heart rate and blood pressure while measuring stress levels through galvanic skin response.

Already Happening (%)	Very Likely (%)	Somewhat Likely (%)	Neutral (%)	Somewhat Unlikely (%)	Very Unlikely (%)
19	31	25	16	6	2

Our organization will use predictive algorithms to facilitate the early treatment of patients' medical problems.

Already Happening (%)	Very Likely (%)	Somewhat Likely (%)	Neutral (%)	Somewhat Unlikely (%)	Very Unlikely (%)
1	10	17	23	27	22

At least half of all surgeries at our organization will be performed with robotics.

Already Happening (%)	Very Likely (%)	Somewhat Likely (%)	Neutral (%)	Somewhat Unlikely (%)	Very Unlikely (%)
1	6	10	21	26	37

Our organization will use drones to deliver medical supplies and perform remote diagnostics for emergency medicine.

Already Happening (%)	Very Likely (%)	Somewhat Likely (%)	Neutral (%)	Somewhat Unlikely (%)	Very Unlikely (%)
6	7	15	22	15	35

Our organization will routinely use brain implant technology to treat conditions such as paralysis, Parkinson's disease and major depression.

Note: Percentages in each row may not sum exactly to 100 percent because of rounding.

What Health Care Executives Anticipate by 2024

- Half of health care executives either already are using predictive algorithms to facilitate the early treatment of patients' medical problems or are very likely to do so.

- Fifty percent of respondents are at least somewhat likely to use "smart clothing" with embedded electronics for patient care.

- Nearly half (49 percent) of leaders think it unlikely that most surgeries at their hospital or health system will be performed using robotics.

—*continued from pg. 17*

a breakdown of the nervous system, such as paralysis.

Bioelectronic medicine, which combines neuroscience with molecular biology and bioengineering, is helping to turn that hope into reality by enabling clinicians to tap into the nervous system through devices that emit and detect electrical impulses. In an effort to invent new and smarter diagnostic and treatment equipment, researchers are learning the language of neural signals to identify and effectively treat diseases and injuries.

Many opportunities exist to further our knowledge and technology development in the field, such as refining neural implants, identifying ways to enhance the reliability and long-term performance of bioelectronics and continued mapping of the human nervous system, to name a few. There also are questions about how the brain and peripheral nervous system communicate, given their sheer size and complexity. Hospitals and health systems can look for ways to get engaged in clinical or laboratory research to help drive the field of bioelectronic medicine forward.

Technological Developments Accelerating Discovery

Recent innovations in data analytics (especially machine learning) are accelerating discoveries and advances in bioelectronic medicine. By analyzing large amounts of data on how the nervous system communicates with the body, researchers can identify signals of both disease and health.

For example, at the Center for Bioelectronic Medicine at the Feinstein Institute, machine learning was a component of recent research that successfully decoded specific neural signals related to inflammation (Zanos et al. 2018). Researchers can use the decoding methods from this study to identify the neural signaling in a variety of other medical conditions. The study's findings can also be used as the basis for the development of devices that employ the latest microchip technology to support the processing power of large amounts of data on something as small as a nerve.

While many of the discoveries published recently are related to implantable devices, innovations in wearable technology will also play a major role in creating new therapies and treatments. As textile-based electronics begin to emerge, "smart clothing" applications will multiply—for example, shirts that monitor heart rate and blood pressure while measuring stress levels through galvanic skin response. In addition to these diagnostic applications, we will see therapeutic and rehabilitation devices that can potentially help with postsurgical and poststroke recovery.

Industry Driving Clinical Trials

The discoveries in the lab are being made possible by investment from industry. Leaders such as Alphabet Inc.'s Verily and GSK (GlaxoSmithKline), which recently partnered to form Galvani Bioelectronics, and other companies such as Medtronic, Teva, Boston Scientific, GE and United Therapeutics recognize this technology as a growing sector that will present alternatives to the biochemical therapies traditionally offered by Big Pharma to treat many diseases and conditions. Therefore, these companies are supporting the development of bioelectronic medicine devices and clinical trials.

Major health care organizations, such as Northwell Health, are also dedicating research funding to the field and conducting clinical trials and translational studies. Discoveries made in the lab can be patented and licensed to outside companies, generating additional revenue for hospitals and health systems.

In fact, the Feinstein Institute's discovery of the inflammatory reflex led to the development of new treatment methods for RA that have been licensed to SetPoint Medical. Initial clinical study findings have been promising. SetPoint recently hosted a clinical trial in Amsterdam that found that active electrical stimulation of the vagus nerve inhibits production of the cell-signaling protein TNF—a key contributor to inflammation in RA patients—and significantly attenuates the severity of the disease (Koopman et al. 2016). As a result, the company launched trials in the United States in 2018 for RA and has supported trials in Europe for Crohn's disease.

Conducting research in a hospital also allows collaboration with clinicians to provide patients with access to cutting-edge care discovered through clinical trials. For example, in a first-of-its-kind study that examined bioelectronic methods in the treatment of traumatic injury, volitional hand movement was restored in a completely paralyzed man through the use of a brain implant. The experimental device decoded brain signals and rerouted them to affected muscles so that movement was regained—through thought alone (Bouton et al. 2016).

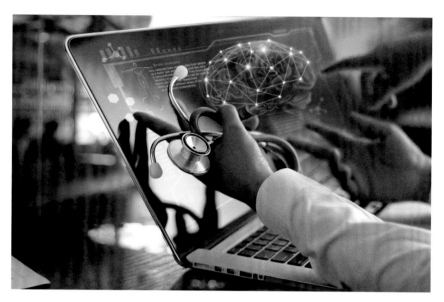

What's in Store for the Future?

As technology and discoveries expand, we can expect rapid growth in the field that could greatly improve how we deliver care. As mentioned, progress is already being made with Crohn's, lupus and RA therapies, and advances in treatments for paralysis may emerge in the near future.

Although it is likely to take time before bioelectronic medicine is used as commonly as pacemakers, a growing number of clinical studies are becoming available. Health professionals need to keep pace with research and advances and be prepared for patient inquiries about whether they are viable for their condition.

If your hospital has a research component, awareness of bioelectronic medicine can also lead to collaborations with other institutions and industry. The research being conducted at your facility has the potential to attract donors and industry investment.

To support the connection to industry while protecting new discoveries, health care leaders should consider dedicating staff to help with patenting. This kind of support provides the foundation for licensing opportunities for the researchers and the health organization.

As with other emerging technologies, providers should encourage discussion about the challenges of bioelectronic medicine and possible ethical questions that may arise. Holding conferences and community events can provide clinicians with the latest information and educate the public on current research. Such efforts will help address concerns and offer insight into clinical studies and treatment options.

As bioelectronic medicine continues to take hold and is proven effective, we may soon see medical professionals reading nervous system signals through either implanted or external devices to diagnose and treat disease. By making it a priority to stay abreast of developments in this arena, hospital and health system executives have the opportunity to collaborate in this research and thereby bring new therapies to their patients and communities sooner.

References

Bouton, C.E., A. Shaikhouni, N.V. Annetta, M.A. Bockbrader, D.A. Friedenberg, D.M. Nielson, G. Sharma, P.B. Sederberg, B.C. Glenn, W.J. Mysiw, A.G. Morgan, M. Deogaonkar and A.R. Rezai. 2016. "Restoring Cortical Control of Functional Movement in a Human with Quadriplegia." *Nature* 533 (7602): 247–50.

Koopman, F.A., S.S. Chavan, S. Miljko, S. Grazio, S. Sokolovic, P.R. Schuurman, A.D. Mehta, Y.A. Levine, M. Faltys, R. Zitnik, K.J. Tracey and P.P. Tak. 2016. "Vagus Nerve Stimulation Inhibits Cytokine Production and Attenuates Disease Severity in Rheumatoid Arthritis." *Proceedings of the National Academy of Sciences of the United States of America* 113 (29): 8284–89.

Tracey, K.J. 2002. "The Inflammatory Reflex." *Nature* 420 (6917): 853–59.

Zanos, T.P., H.A. Silverman, T. Levy, T. Tsaava, E. Battinelli, P.W. Lorraine, J.M. Ashe, S.S. Chavan, K.J. Tracey and C.E. Bouton. 2018. "Identification of Cytokine-Specific Sensory Neural Signals by Decoding Murine Vagus Nerve Activity." *Proceedings of the National Academy of Sciences of the United States of America* 115 (21): E4843–52.

Adopting the Attributes of High-Value Hospitals

by David S.P. Hopkins, Ph.D., Melora Simon, Thomas Wang, Ph.D., and Arnold Milstein, M.D.

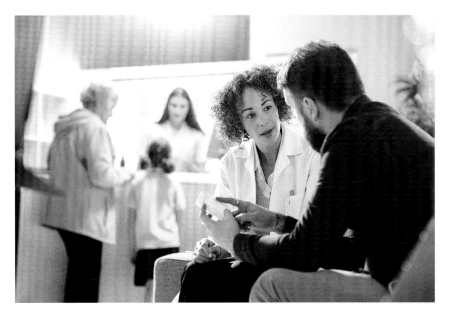

Hospital care in the United States continues to move, albeit fitfully, toward value-based payment models driven in large part by the Centers for Medicare & Medicaid Services (CMS). The purpose of value-based payment is to reduce annual per capita and per-episode costs to payers and patients and improve the quality of care (Bannow 2018). In addition, private purchasers are more actively opposing the pricing practices of large hospitals and health systems by encouraging patients to select higher-value hospitals through narrow networks and reference pricing, supporting antitrust initiatives, lobbying for no-surprise balance billing laws and other means.

To help hospitals respond constructively, Stanford University's Clinical Excellence Research Center undertook the America's Most Valuable Care study, which was supported by the Peterson Center on Healthcare (2018). The study used positive outlier research methods to identify "bright spots" among community hospitals, both large and small, that consistently deliver high-quality care at a low total per-episode cost on measures of value used by private payers. The study revealed attributes of care delivery that separate these hospitals from their

About the Authors

David S.P. Hopkins, Ph.D., is research advisor at the Clinical Excellence Research Center (CERC) at Stanford University. Prior to joining CERC, he served as director of quality measurement and improvement at the Pacific Business Group on Health. Earlier in his career, he was director of corporate affiliations and policy at Stanford University Hospital. Hopkins received his master of science degree in statistics and his doctorate in operations research from Stanford University.

Melora Simon leads the California Quality Collaborative, a statewide multistakeholder collaborative to reengineer health care. Previously, she was the director of America's Most Valuable Care initiative at CERC. Simon holds a master's degree in health services management from Columbia University and a bachelor of arts degree in human biology from Stanford University.

Thomas Wang, Ph.D., is the director of health insights at Cardinal Analytx, a health care startup. Earlier in his career, he served in various roles with health care organizations including CERC and Nuna Health. Wang has a background in health and organizational economics and received his doctorate in economics from Harvard University.

Arnold Milstein, M.D., is a professor of medicine at Stanford University and directs CERC, which develops scalable innovations in clinical process and in bedside applications of machine intelligence that lower the cost of high-quality health care. Before joining Stanford's faculty, he created and globalized a health care performance improvement firm; cofounded three nationally influential public benefit initiatives, including The Leapfrog Group; served as a congressional Medicare Payment Advisory Commission commissioner; and was elected to the National Academy of Medicine.

FUTURESCAN SURVEY RESULTS
Value-Based Care

How likely is it that the following will happen by 2024?

Already Happening (%)	Very Likely (%)	Somewhat Likely (%)	Neutral (%)	Somewhat Unlikely (%)	Very Unlikely (%)
18	32	29	14	5	3

Our organization will increase, by at least 20 percent, its fiscal investment in population health strategies to address social determinants of health.

Already Happening (%)	Very Likely (%)	Somewhat Likely (%)	Neutral (%)	Somewhat Unlikely (%)	Very Unlikely (%)
19	27	30	13	9	3

Our organization will purchase or establish a joint venture with a primary care entity that has an explicit mission to reduce inpatient days and intensive outpatient procedures and replace them with more coaching, in-home and virtual outreach, and other primary care services.

Already Happening (%)	Very Likely (%)	Somewhat Likely (%)	Neutral (%)	Somewhat Unlikely (%)	Very Unlikely (%)
10	24	34	16	9	7

Our organization will at least double its investment in addressing social determinants of health in our region, such as improving housing access, improving the built environment (e.g., parks, recreating or walkability), outreach to teenagers around education/crime reduction and improving access to fresh food.

Already Happening (%)	Very Likely (%)	Somewhat Likely (%)	Neutral (%)	Somewhat Unlikely (%)	Very Unlikely (%)
17	26	26	12	14	4

To reduce the need for hospital admissions, our organization's emergency department staff will have access to case managers with the authority to pay for a defined set of interventions, including nonhealthcare and nonreimbursable interventions such as temporary housing.

Already Happening (%)	Very Likely (%)	Somewhat Likely (%)	Neutral (%)	Somewhat Unlikely (%)	Very Unlikely (%)
13	35	26	16	8	2

Unit leaders will have access to staff to identify and remove nonclinical obstacles (e.g., insecure housing, domestic abuse or insufficient access to prescriptions) so the patient can be released when clinically ready.

Already Happening (%)	Very Likely (%)	Somewhat Likely (%)	Neutral (%)	Somewhat Unlikely (%)	Very Unlikely (%)
	66	23	9	2	0 0

Our organization will hold all staff accountable to intervene whenever they observe a situation that violates patient safety protocol (e.g., skipping a checklist set or closing a surgical incision before sponge counts are confidently reconciled).

continued on pg. 23

—continued from pg. 21

peers. Many bright-spot hospitals operate independently of major health systems that have the advantage of large scale or unique medical cultures formed over decades. The findings apply to most nonrural, nonacademic community hospitals and health systems.

Three Types of High-Value Attributes

Three major themes characterize attributes of care that distinguish hospitals ranking favorably on clinical and financial outcomes valued by payers.

Thinking beyond the hospital stay. High-value hospitals hold themselves accountable for ensuring the successful transition of inpatients from hospital to home well beyond 30 days. They identify patients who have a higher likelihood of readmission and send members of the care team to conduct home visits or provide

additional support to skilled nursing facilities (SNFs). They also invest in palliative care programs to help ensure that the care provided is consistent with patients' values and goals.

Example: One study hospital established strong relationships with a few select local SNFs. Rapid and efficient communication between the entities facilitated the transfer of patients to the SNFs, including in some cases direct admissions from the emergency department (ED). The hospital provided deeper support to these select SNFs by placing its own employed clinical staff at the facilities.

Cutting waste, not safety. High-value hospitals reduce the cost of care in two distinct ways. One is by decreasing the unnecessary spending that occurs when low-acuity patients are cared for in an inappropriate setting (e.g., the ED or intensive care unit) or when they stay in the hospital for longer than needed. The other is through efficient management (e.g., of supplies

continued from pg. 22

| 39 | 27 | 17 | 10 | 6 | 1 |

Unit staffing at our organization will be assessed multiple times daily to ensure that no unit is understaffed for more than one hour.

| 18 | 24 | 25 | 21 | 6 | 5 |

For some complex surgeries, an established threshold of volume is associated with better outcomes. Our organization will not perform these surgeries unless (a) the surgery is an emergency or (b) our organization has already achieved such volume.

Note: Percentages in each row may not sum exactly to 100 percent because of rounding.

What Health Care Executives Anticipate by 2024

- Nearly eight in 10 respondents (79 percent) indicate their organization is at least somewhat likely to increase its fiscal investment in population health strategies by 20 percent or more to address social determinants of health.

- Two-thirds of health care executives already hold all staff accountable to intervene when they see a patient safety concern. Another 23 percent are very likely to do so.

- Sixty-eight percent of leaders are at least somewhat likely to double the investment in addressing social determinants of health.

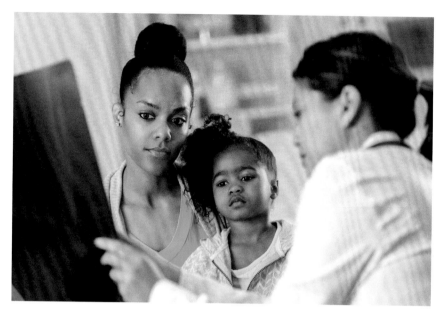

—continued from pg. 23

and staff) to minimize expenditures and attain high quality.

Example: A hospital actively manages patient flow through the use of a program known as "real-time demand management," which has several components. The first consists of twice-daily, rapid-fire bed meetings in which clinical unit leaders and other involved staff (e.g., case managers and social workers) identify obstacles to discharge and focus nurse managers on clearing critical care beds before 2 p.m., when ED admissions rise. In addition, each unit predicts the number of discharges by time of day, as well as likely admissions of patients currently in the ED or coming from surgery, and tracks their predictive accuracy over time. During the past year, accuracy has risen from 30 percent to nearly 85 percent, and average length of stay has decreased by half a day. Essentially, the staff have become more attentive to the discharge process and much better at estimating—and planning for—eventual discharge.

Engaging the frontline team in improving the cost-effectiveness of needed care. High-value hospitals commonly demonstrate the following:

- Staff are utilized to their fullest potential, both in enhancing the care provided and in supporting other team members.

- The opinions of staff are respected and seen as critical to improving quality and safety.
- Physicians are engaged in multiple aspects of the hospital, often serving in leadership positions and holding their peers to higher quality standards.
- Staff in various positions are maximally utilized to relieve clinicians of some burdens and responsibilities.

Example: One hospital has fully incorporated the principles of Team-STEPPS (an evidence-based team communication system designed to enhance patient safety) and Just Culture (an organizational culture in which front-line staff are not punished for actions, omissions or decisions commensurate with their experience and training, but conscious disregard of clear risks to patients and gross misconduct are not tolerated). As a result, its staff clearly display a commitment to patient safety. For instance, nurses do not allow a surgical procedure to proceed if the surgical checklist is not complete. The hospital's leaders wholeheartedly embrace the value of nonhierarchical communication for patient safety. Leaders and staff alike place great importance on Team-STEPPS communication frameworks and acknowledge the obligation to dissent when an unjustified deviation from intended care is detected.

Futurescan Survey Results

The *Futurescan* national survey of health care leaders included tracer questions focused on a small set of care delivery attributes commonly exhibited by community hospitals that rank favorably on payer measures of quality and cost per hospital episode of care.

Because most hospitals do not participate in accountable care organization (ACO) programs that reward decreases in preventable hospital admissions (other than readmissions within 30 days of hospital discharge), we hypothesized that hospitals are adopting attributes likely to improve value per episode rather than tactics aimed at reducing preventable admissions. We also speculated that care delivery attributes that reduce high-revenue treatments (e.g., complex elective surgeries) are the least widely adopted.

In addition, the *Futurescan* survey included questions that examined hospitals' progress toward adopting attributes to improve quality and reduce cost per episode of care, items designed to probe whether hospitals are taking action to reduce preventable admissions, and one tracer question to determine whether hospitals are implementing practices that would improve value but depress high-revenue services.

As expected, attributes that aim to improve the quality of inpatient episodes while reducing costs have gained (and will likely continue to gain) near-term adoption. In particular, the emphasis by CMS and other major payers on eliminating reimbursement for patient safety failures appears to be paying off (Blumenthal, Abrams and Nuzum 2015). A notable exception is that few hospitals ensure that unit leaders have the resources needed to remove nonclinical obstacles to discharge, suggesting that hospitals do not yet fully understand how they can cost-effectively address social determinants of health and mitigate preventable health care utilization.

With respect to attributes requiring a greater focus on population health management, we observe a different result. Although only 18 percent of respondents indicated that they have increased investment in population health strategies to address social determinants of health, more than 60 percent said they are at least somewhat likely to do so in the next five years. Clearly, continued encouragement of ACOs by CMS and other payers is having an impact on hospital strategic planning for near-term improvement in the value of all services provided to patients who predominantly receive care at a particular hospital.

Finally, one action included in the *Futurescan* survey that is likely to improve quality while imposing large per-episode revenue losses stands out as the least widely implemented (or least likely to be implemented in the near future). Fewer than half of respondents indicated that redirecting patients who require complex surgeries for which their hospital lacks sufficient experience is already happening or is very likely to happen by 2024. This result is not surprising; low-volume hospitals are loath to antagonize admitting physicians or lose substantial incremental revenue from complex elective procedures, despite evidence of increased risk of treatment complications if annual volume fails to meet scientifically determined minimum thresholds.

of care). Our study and the *Futurescan* survey found much slower adoption of strategies likely to prevent admissions. Stronger payer incentives may be required to accelerate adoption of attributes that reduce occupancy. As payers gradually increase rewards for yearlong excellence in care delivery, hospital and

---

Hospital and health system leaders will benefit from implementing best practices and bright spots in value-driven performance that meet the needs of patients and health insurers alike.

Conclusion

Hospitals are rapidly adopting attributes of their high-value peers in areas where they have the greatest economic incentive (e.g., readmissions and episodes health system leaders will benefit from implementing best practices and bright spots in value-driven performance that meet the needs of patients and health insurers alike.

References

Bannow, T. 2018. "Hospitals 'Can't Afford Not to' Provide Value-Based Care." *Modern Healthcare*. Published July 2. www.modernhealthcare.com/article/20180702/NEWS/180709991.

Blumenthal, D., M. Abrams and R. Nuzum. 2015. "The Affordable Care Act at 5 Years." *New England Journal of Medicine* 372 (25): 2451–58.

Peterson Center on Healthcare. 2018. "Uncovering America's Most Valuable Care." Accessed August 4. https://petersonhealthcare.org/identification-uncovering-americas-most-valuable-care.

Health Systems Partner to Grow Consumer-Driven Physician Networks

by Amir Dan Rubin

As the delivery of medical care continues to shift to the outpatient arena, the latest *Futurescan* national survey reveals the torrent pace at which health care organizations are aligning with doctors.

Indeed, 76 percent of responding hospital and health system leaders indicate that they are growing their physician networks by more than 25 percent or are likely to do so by 2024. Primary care doctors have persisted in joining medical groups and health systems, with independent practices declining more than 6 percentage points between 2010 and 2016 to 35 percent of the overall total (Mathews 2018). In less than a decade, the proportion of health system revenues from outpatient services has risen from 28 percent to 47 percent (American Hospital Association 2017).

Physician Aggregation Is Key

The importance of physician aggregation to health care organizations is highlighted by *Futurescan* survey results showing that 75 percent of participants are operating their network at a loss or are willing to do so to achieve broader strategic objectives. Findings from *Modern Healthcare*'s annual Hospital Systems Survey similarly reflect the significance of network development, with 22 percent of

respondents indicating that physician hiring in the prior year had already improved their organization's overall financial performance despite losses incurred on their physician practices (Bannow 2018).

Health systems are pursuing these investments to achieve the following outcomes:

- Align more attributable lives with their networks.
- Deliver higher levels of service, access and value-based care to consumers, employers and payers.
- Prevent providers and their associated patient bases from becoming aligned with competing networks.

To expand their networks, health systems are pursuing a number of approaches, including "making" a network by launching medical groups and medical foundations, buying physician practices and hospitals and constructing medical office buildings and outpatient centers. Such approaches tend to require significant investments in acquisitions, equipment, facilities, technology, operations and management. Aligning priorities and expenditures for these initiatives can be challenging for most health systems because of limited capital and competition from higher-margin inpatient services and

About the Author

Amir Dan Rubin is president and CEO of One Medical, a leading modernized primary care organization that is transforming health care with its innovative member-based, technology-powered model. Previously, he served as executive vice president of UnitedHealth Group's Optum division, where he focused on making the health system work better for everyone. He also was president and CEO of Stanford Health Care—the academic health system affiliated with Stanford University—where he helped raise patient experience and quality scores to the highest levels in the nation, grow a regional physician network and advance digital and population health. Rubin also previously served as chief operating officer (COO) of UCLA Health, as COO of Stony Brook University's health system, as assistant vice president of Memorial Hermann Health System, and as a management consultant at APM Consulting. Rubin holds M.B.A. and M.H.S.A. degrees from the University of Michigan and a B.A. from the University of California, Berkeley, and he has been a recipient of the Ernst & Young Entrepreneur of the Year Award.

Physician Aggregation

How likely is it that the following will happen by 2024?

Already Happening (%)	Very Likely (%)	Somewhat Likely (%)	Neutral (%)	Somewhat Unlikely (%)	Very Unlikely (%)
21	33	22	8	11	6

Our organization will expand our physician network by more than 25 percent.

	Very Likely (%)	Somewhat Likely (%)	Neutral (%)	Somewhat Unlikely (%)	Very Unlikely (%)
	46	13	16	13	8	4

Our organization will be willing to operate our physician network at a loss to achieve broader strategic objectives.

Already Happening (%)	Very Likely (%)	Somewhat Likely (%)	Neutral (%)	Somewhat Unlikely (%)	Very Unlikely (%)
6	44	24	10	12	4

Our organization will face competition for commercially insured patients from new, national market entrants focused on consumerism, such as Google, Apple or Amazon.

	Very Likely (%)	Somewhat Likely (%)	Neutral (%)	Somewhat Unlikely (%)	Very Unlikely (%)
42	34	12	8	3	1

Our organization will pursue external relationships to advance our physician network and better serve consumer demands (e.g., through partnerships for consumer-driven primary care, employer clinics, virtual care, urgent care or retail care).

Already Happening (%)	Very Likely (%)	Somewhat Likely (%)	Neutral (%)	Somewhat Unlikely (%)	Very Unlikely (%)
25	43	21	10	1	1

Our organization will have established new physician network models, partnerships and technology to reduce physician burnout.

Note: Percentages in each row may not sum exactly to 100 percent because of rounding.

What Health Care Executives Anticipate by 2024

- Nearly half (46 percent) of hospital and health system executives are already operating their physician network at a loss to achieve broader strategic objectives. Another 29 percent are at least somewhat likely to do so.

- A clear majority (76 percent) of leaders already are pursuing or are very likely to pursue external relationships to advance their physician network and better serve consumers.

- Eighty-nine percent of responding health care executives are at least somewhat likely to establish new physician network models and partnerships or to use technology solutions to reduce doctor burnout.

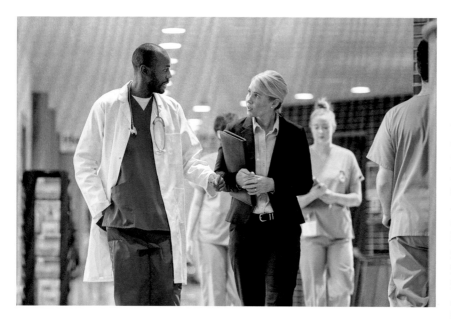

—continued from pg. 26

procedural care that still serve as cash cows.

Other network development strategies include contractual alignment models such as clinically integrated networks (CINs), independent practice associations (IPAs) and provider-sponsored or joint-venture health plans. Although these options can mean less up-front funding for bricks and mortar, they typically demand substantial investments in leadership, technology and risk-based capital. To be most impactful, they may also require riskier contractual arrangements with significant downside and upside financial risk, as well as sizeable ongoing investments to achieve broader strategic aims.

Physician aggregation strategies involving ownership, acquisition or affiliation can also face structural challenges in addressing consumer needs and value-based objectives. Indeed, health systems' embedded fee-for-service payment models and electronic health record (EHR) systems are often more aligned to volume-driven and episodic care than to continuous digital engagement and relationship-based care. Some organizations intentionally segment their various business-line strategies to try to disentangle these sometimes conflicting economic and technology requirements. For example, during my time as president and CEO of Stanford Health Care in

California, the health system developed distinct approaches for its complex care, network of care, population care and digital care segments.

The market is also seeing new ambulatory care entrants innovating to deliver higher levels of service and access to meet the rising expectations of consumers and employers. Such entrants can more nimbly develop customized technology and realigned economic models without being encumbered by the complexities of running entire hospitals or health systems. They often can take advantage of private capital pools not typically available to nonprofit or even publicly traded organizations. As a result, health systems are also partnering with innovators to offer tailored network solutions to distinct customer segments, draw on additional capital pools while managing investment risks and further extend the reach as well as protect the draw of their networks.

Futurescan survey results show that 74 percent of responding health care leaders believe new market entrants are now competing (or are likely to compete) with them for their most profitable, commercially insured patients if they do not pursue partnerships. A 2017 marketplace survey of executives, clinical leaders and clinicians similarly revealed that 54 percent of survey participants believe that disruptive innovation for hospitals and health systems will come

from startups, and 36 percent consider primary care to be the health care sector most in need of disruptive innovation (Dafny and Mohta 2017).

Employers and consumers with commercial insurance who are frustrated with the current state of health care are directly calling for new and innovative approaches. According to a 2018 National Business Group on Health survey, 70 percent of employers believe new entrants are necessary to disrupt the market in a positive way. Meanwhile, businesses continue to see commercial insurance premiums outpace general inflation by more than 4 percent (Tracer 2017). Additionally, more than 50 percent of physicians show symptoms of burnout in the current system, driven in part by fee-for-service productivity demands, rising insurance system complexities and EHR burdens (Shanafelt et al. 2015). As a result, doctors are looking for alternatives to both traditional independent practices and hospital-based alignment.

A Trend Toward Partnerships

Increasingly, hospitals and health systems are acknowledging that trying to meet the evolving needs of consumers, employers and physicians on their own might be an insufficient strategy, particularly given the speed of change in the marketplace and the investments and focus required to be successful. Accordingly, they are finding that partnering with innovators can prove to be an effective and targeted way to serve employers and consumers who have the highest level of choice. Innovative partners can often develop aligned networks faster and at a lower cost and can integrate them directly into health care organizations through affiliations.

A full 88 percent of *Futurescan* survey respondents indicate a willingness to pursue external relationships to advance their networks and better accommodate consumer demands for services such as primary care, employer clinics, virtual care, urgent care and retail care. Results show that 42 percent of executives have already entered into these types of partnerships, and another 34 percent are highly likely to do so in the next five years.

For example, health systems have been developing relationships with large primary care groups such as One Medical (where I serve as president and CEO) to further advance their networks through innovative direct-to-employer and consumer-driven strategies while minimizing their capital expenditures, business risk and time to market. Providers have also pursued network-extending relationships with operators of urgent care centers, surgery centers, freestanding emergency departments, diagnostic testing facilities, telehealth companies and drugstore retail clinics.

These partnerships and affiliations may take a variety of forms, including professional service and management service agreements, lease arrangements, joint ventures, CINs, cost-plus contracts, fee-for-service and salaried physician models, IPA relationships and capitated or accountable care organization–like arrangements. Many health care organizations also find that these options can spread capital burdens and business risks as all partners commit resources and management energy.

Successful physician aggregation partnerships require alignment on goals, thoughtful assessments, fair contractual terms and ongoing relationship management. They should be built on both mutual success and mutual trust. Key issues for hospital and health system leaders to consider when evaluating potential partnerships include the following:

- **Strategy:** How well aligned are the objectives and strategies of the two organizations?
- **Market impact:** Does the partner allow the hospital or health system to improve its position in the market

with consumers, employers, payers and other stakeholders?
- **Competitors:** Will the partner offer exclusivity and thus a marketplace advantage to the hospital or health system?
- **Differentiation:** Does the partner bring any differentiators to the table in terms of offerings, speed to market, market positioning, technology, attributable lives, consumer

---

Health systems will increasingly deploy a composite of owned, leased and partnership-based networks.

---

engagement, employer relationships, provider alignment or other factors?
- **Economic models:** Are there aligned opportunities for financial success?
- **Capital and business risk:** Does the partner help preserve capital and deflect financial or business risk away from the health care organization?
- **Operational:** Does the partner relieve the provider of any administrative burdens? How will operational coordination occur?
- **Technology:** Does the partner bring innovative technology that is compelling to consumers, employers, providers and payers?
- **Stickiness:** How enduring or lasting will the relationship be, and how much does this matter?

Conclusion

The *Futurescan* survey demonstrates the continued strong movement by health systems to implement physician aggregation and network expansion strategies.

Indeed, outpatient income now accounts for almost half of all hospital and health system revenues, prompting leaders to pursue an array of options to better serve the needs of consumers and employers.

The survey results indicate that health care organizations persist in building their networks through owned, leased, acquired, employed and affiliated medical group models. These approaches require significant and thoughtful invest-ments in capital, technology, operations and leadership. They also involve a nuanced adaptation of payer reimbursement models, compensation and EHRs.

The survey also reveals the large role played by a variety of partnerships in network development as health systems seek to extend their reach, deliver high-value care and advance growth in attributable lives. Moreover, partnerships can diffuse business risks, preserve capital and defend against competitors and disruptors. Beneficial partnerships are built on strong alignment of strategic, financial and operational factors. They require up-front development and ongoing management.

In light of the survey's findings that health systems will increasingly deploy a composite of owned, leased and partnership-based networks, organizational and leadership roles, competencies and structures will need to evolve to support successful enterprise management in the future.

References

American Hospital Association. 2017. "2018 Environmental Scan." *Hospitals & Health Networks*. Published October. www.hhnmag.com/ext/resources/inc-hhn/pdfs/Environmental-Scan-2018/ES18_complete_with_ads.pdf.

Bannow, T. 2018. "Docs Don't Drain Hospital Finances, Systems Say." *Modern Healthcare*. Published July 14. www.modernhealthcare.com/article/20180714/NEWS/180719978.

Dafny, L., and S. Mohta. 2017. "New Marketplace Survey: The Sources of Health Care Innovation." *NEJM Catalyst*. Published February 16. https://catalyst.nejm.org/disruptive-innovation-in-healthcare-survey/.

Mathews, A.W. 2018. "Behind Your Rising Health-Care Bills: Secret Hospital Deals That Squelch Competition." *Wall Street Journal*. Published September 18. www.wsj.com/articles/behind-your-rising-health-care-bills-secret-hospital-deals-that-squelch-competition-1537281963.

National Business Group on Health. 2018. "2019 Large Employers' Health Care Strategy and Plan Design Survey." Published August 7. www.businessgrouphealth.org/pub/B7F87411-A59D-D212-CA59-2A79A7683DF2.

Shanafelt, T.D., O. Hasan, L.N. Dyrbye, C. Sinsky, D. Satale, J. Sloan and C.P. West. 2015. "Changes in Burnout and Satisfaction with Work–Life Balance in Physicians and the General US Working Population Between 2011 and 2014." *Mayo Clinic Proceedings* 90 (12): 1600–1613.

Tracer, Z. 2017. "Rising Health-Insurance Costs Are Eating into Employees' Paycheck Gains." Bloomberg. Published September 19. www.bloomberg.com/news/articles/2017-09-19/rising-health-insurance-costs-blunt-employees-paycheck-gains.

Reaching the Limits of the Governance Model

by James E. Orlikoff

Effective governance of hospitals and health systems is challenging and will only become more so. Efforts to address these challenges usually have focused on elevating governance to "best practice" levels. Although this approach is appropriate (and necessary), it is insufficient in the face of growing obstacles and the emergence of new, more systemic threats to our longtime governance model. Today's governance challenges require disruption of the traditional model and the creation of updated ones that are more relevant to the new environment.

The traditional governance model goes back to the founding of the first U.S. hospital in 1751 by Benjamin Franklin and Thomas Bond, and it has endured largely unchanged to this day. This model has several basic, implicit components that are largely taken for granted, including community-based governance; a tolerance for conflicts of interest that serve community relationships; diffuse and variable accountability of both boards and board members; and long-tenured, uncompensated (volunteer) trustees who make only a minimal time commitment and lack standardized training (Orlikoff 2018).

This traditional model can no longer be taken for granted because it is

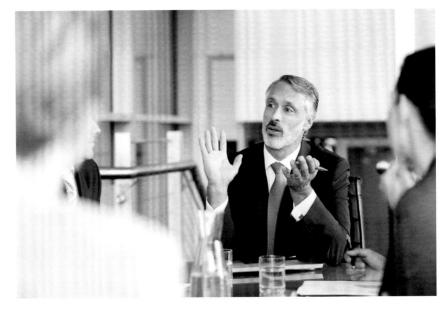

straining under the pressures of its age and two significant categories of trends. The first is the rapidly changing and radically challenging health care landscape, which includes—but is certainly not limited to—relentless downward financial pressures, consolidation and growth of supersystems, disruptive competition and consumerism. To this familiar litany must be added two challenges specific to governance: (1) the growing burden of regulatory and legal requirements placed on health care boards and (2) the increasing complexity of governance's

very structure and function, especially in increasingly large health care systems.

As daunting as the first category is, it is the second that portends the obsolescence of the traditional model of health care governance: namely, the sweeping scope of broad societal change brought about by economic, demographic, generational and cultural forces.

Demographics: Boards Are Aging

As society struggles with an aging population and narrowing ratios of young

About the Author

James E. Orlikoff is president of Orlikoff & Associates Inc., a Chicago-based consulting firm specializing in health care governance and leadership, strategy, and quality and safety. He is the national advisor on governance and leadership to the American Hospital Association. Orlikoff has advised hospitals and systems in 12 countries and has worked extensively with U.S. hospital and system governing boards to strengthen their overall effectiveness and oversight of strategy and quality. The author of 15 books and more than a hundred articles, he has served on hospital, health system, college and civic boards. He is currently a member of the St. Charles Health System board in Bend, Oregon. He is an author of *Board Work: Governing Health Care Organizations* (Jossey-Bass, 1999), which won the American College of Healthcare Executives James A. Hamilton Book of the Year Award in 2000.

Governance

How likely is it that the following will happen by 2024?

Already Happening (%)	Very Likely (%)	Somewhat Likely (%)	Neutral (%)	Somewhat Unlikely (%)	Very Unlikely (%)
16	21	14	19	17	13

Recruiting and retaining qualified board members will be one of the three most significant challenges for our organization's governing board.

| 27 | 25 | 19 | 14 | 10 | 4 |

Our organization will have a strategic goal to increase the generational diversity of our governing board.

| 14 | 9 | 16 | 20 | 20 | 21 |

Our organization will increasingly seek board members who live and work outside our service area.

| 5 | 6 | 6 | 14 | 28 | 40 |

Our organization will compensate board members, beyond reimbursement of expenses.

| 1 | 14 | 19 | 29 | 24 | 13 |

Our organization will change governance models to attract and retain millennials.

Note: Percentages in each row may not sum exactly to 100 percent because of rounding.

What Health Care Executives Anticipate by 2024

- About half (51 percent) of respondents indicate that recruiting and retaining qualified board members will be one of their three top challenges for organizational governance.

- Twenty-seven percent of leaders say they already have a strategic goal to increase the generational diversity of their hospital or health system governing board. Another 44 percent are at least somewhat likely to establish such a goal.

- More than a third (34 percent) of respondents say they have changed their organizational governing model to attract millennials or are at least somewhat likely to do so.

—continued from pg. 31

to old, so does governance. Health care boards are getting older. Since 2005, the percentage of board members under the age of 50 has declined. In 2005, respondents to a national governance survey of CEOs and board chairs of freestanding hospitals, subsidiary hospitals and health systems reported that 29 percent of their board's members were aged 50 or younger. In 2011, that figure decreased to 24 percent, and by 2014 it had dropped to 21 percent. More significantly, respondents from health systems reported that only 12 percent of their board's members were aged 50 or younger in 2014 (American Hospital Association Center for Healthcare Governance 2014). Health care leaders responding to the latest *Futurescan* national survey clearly recognize this challenge:

- Twenty-seven percent reported that they already have a strategic goal to increase generational diversity on their boards.
- Twenty-five percent said they are very likely to do so in the next five years.
- Nineteen percent stated they are somewhat likely to do so.

Baby boomers will not be able to serve as the primary generational pool of health care board members much longer. Yet, anecdotal reports from hospital and health system executives and board members suggest they are having difficulty recruiting and retaining millennials and Gen Xers as board members. Although this difficulty may be the result of half-hearted or misguided recruitment efforts, it is also possible that younger generations have different views on volunteerism or are not able to make the significant time commitment that governance increasingly requires.

Economics and Society: Who Has the Time?

Time demands on health care board members are growing and are an increasing cause of complaint. Many CEOs and board chairs report that their meetings now last longer than in the recent past. Others say they have added new committees that consume more of board members' and executives' time. For example, "the prevalence of a standing quality committee has markedly increased in the last decade; fewer than six in 10 boards reported having a quality committee in 2005, compared to more than eight in 10 boards reporting a quality

committee in 2014" (American Hospital Association Center for Healthcare Governance 2014, 17).

Further, a robust continuing governance education process is widely considered to be a best practice for board members to keep up with the dizzying changes in the health care environment and the implications for their hospitals and health systems. Yet, despite its growing importance, continuing governance education demands even more time of volunteer trustees. Perhaps that is why participation by board members is declining and why nearly all types of board education decreased from 2011 to 2014 (American Hospital Association Center for Healthcare Governance 2014). Board members likely find the time demands of education excessive and unacceptable, especially Gen Xers and millennials who are busy building careers and raising families.

Consider this excerpt from an email that was sent to me in July 2017 by a Gen X member of a health system board who is an accomplished executive and the mother of several young children:

Hi Jamie: Hope you are doing well. I wanted to speak with you regarding the [health system] board. By way of background, I sit on a number of other boards, and the [health system] board and committees take up as much time as all the other three put together. I am considering early resignation from the board due to this and the fact that I don't feel "aligned" with the organization.

This individual possessed the expertise and demographic characteristics that the health system board fervently desired, but she ultimately resigned well before her term expired. This particular health system did not demand extreme amounts of time from its board members relative to other health systems, yet it consumed "as much time as all the other three" corporate boards she served on "put together." What is it about health system governance that requires triple the time commitment of for-profit, corporate boards? More importantly, is this kind of time demand on volunteer trustees sustainable?

The question is even more acute in the context of other societal trends, such as the shrinking middle class, the 24/7 world of business and a "gig" economy that requires flexible schedules and challenges volunteers' commitments to board meetings and retreats regardless of how far in advance they are booked.

Implications for Health Care Leaders

With the traditional health care governance model under growing and unsustainable pressure, leaders can expect a number of changes in the near future.

Recruiting and retaining qualified board members will become more difficult. This difficulty will have many causes, in particular the expanding complexity of governance, increasing time demands and growing concern about exposure to reputational risk and liability. Whatever the cause, this challenge is already perceived by a slim majority of *Futurescan* survey respondents: 16 percent indicated they are already experiencing difficulty in recruiting and retaining board members, and 35 percent stated it is somewhat to very likely recruitment and retention will become problematic by 2024. Interestingly, 30 percent of respondents believe it somewhat to very unlikely that recruitment and retention will be challenging, and 19 percent were neutral.

The average age of board members will continue to increase, and age diversity will become a growing issue. An overwhelming majority of the health care leaders participating in the *Futurescan* survey recognize this problem: 71 percent responded that they already have a goal to increase generational diversity on their board or are somewhat to very likely to have such a goal in the next five years. Yet, the future impact of this trend and the possible need to develop new governance models to address it is clearly not accepted: Only 1 percent of respondents said their organizations are already changing their governance models to attract millennials, and just 33 percent said they are somewhat to very likely to do so in the near future.

Effective integration of millennials and Gen Xers into current governance models will be a greater challenge. Hospitals and health systems that have successfully recruited millennials and Gen Xers to their boards frequently report challenges in creating a common,

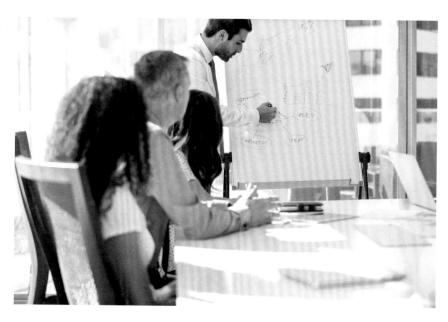

productive governance culture. These challenges are often attributed to a generational culture clash, as millennials and Gen Xers supposedly have radically different approaches than their boomer elders to fulfilling commitments to attend board and committee meetings and using technology during and between meetings. They also tend to lack experience in group dynamics and have a low tolerance for ambiguity and the diffuse, time-consuming governance decision-making processes that result from it.

Leaders will experiment with new governance approaches. As executives and board chairs increasingly struggle to squeeze diminishing functional benefit from the current governance model, they will likely first attempt to make the model work by using approaches seemingly antithetical to it. An example is the practice of appointing a few individuals to the board who live and work well outside the hospital's or health system's service area to gain independent perspectives and rare expertise. Although doing so is a well-known best practice in governance, it is alien to the traditional model, which holds that governance on behalf of a community necessitates governance exclusively by members of that community. Perhaps for this reason, only 14 percent of *Futurescan* survey respondents reported that their

organizations currently seek board members who live and work outside their service area, and just 25 percent indicated this is somewhat to very likely to happen by 2024.

Similarly, although it is not currently considered a best practice, compensation of board members is a possible strategy to address many of the challenges to the traditional governance model, especially the time commitment. However, this idea is so antithetical to one of the basic concepts of the traditional model (voluntary board service) that it was unthinkable to the majority of hospital and health system leaders responding to the *Futurescan* survey. Only 5 percent currently compensate board members, and just 12 percent said they are somewhat to very likely to do so in the next five years.

Failure to aggressively adopt best practices will simply accelerate the collapse of the traditional governance model. Yet, many boards refuse to adopt even well-proven practices that are far less controversial than outside members or compensation. Such practices include reducing the number of boards and committees in a system, practicing competency-based board composition, conducting individual board member performance evaluations pursuant to term renewal, requiring participation in a defined continuing governance education curriculum as a condition for term renewal, and establishing term limits for the board and committee chairs, to name just a few.

Thinking About New Models of Governance

As the traditional model of governance nears the end of its useful life, we must begin to conceptualize and then to experiment with new models that are relevant to a radically different future. One such model could be paid, professional boards composed of outside, independent trustees who are certified experts in health care governance and who contractually agree to fulfill defined time commitments. Another could be the adoption of a common, for-profit model of corporate governance with much smaller boards composed of more insiders and a few outside experts drawn from national searches, all of whom would receive significant compensation. There are many possible future governance models, but they cannot be fully imagined until the implicit rules and rationales for the traditional model are made explicit, along with its profound limits.

Don Berwick said, "Leaders must emerge who regard themselves as

---

Today's governance challenges require disruption of the traditional model and the creation of updated ones that are more relevant to the new environment.

---

defenders not of organizations but of the underlying purposes that have temporarily created those organizations in their current forms. Leaders will have to be willing to unmake the very organizations they hold in trust. That's a big job. It requires a kind of courage that is rare among human beings, including organizational leaders" (Berwick 1992). As the coming crisis in the traditional governance model threatens the very health care system it is tasked with leading, executives and board leaders now face another, even more daunting challenge: to unmake the very models they use to govern before they fail, and then to create new ones that are better suited to lead hospitals and health systems into the future.

References

American Hospital Association Center for Healthcare Governance. 2014. *2014 National Health Care Governance Survey Report*. Chicago: American Hospital Association.

Berwick, D.M. 1992. "Seeking Systemness." *Healthcare Forum Journal* 35 (2): 22–28.

Orlikoff, J. 2018. "Time for a New Model of Governance." *Trustee Insights*. Published July. http://trustees.aha.org/transforminggovernance/articles/time-for-a-new-model-of-governance.shtml.

The Future Role of States in Health Care Policy and Regulation

by Erin C. Fuse Brown, J.D.

Nearly a decade after the passage of the federal Affordable Care Act (ACA), states once again have a growing role in setting health policy and regulating the health care field. Political gridlock has hindered the federal government from moving forward with national reforms, while a renewed emphasis on state flexibility means states are stepping into the vacuum to address a variety of issues.

For states, rising health care costs translate to increasing budgetary pressure in their Medicaid, Children's Health Insurance Program, state employee health coverage, and mental health and substance abuse programs. Increased costs also affect other state health priorities, including access to care in rural areas and the burden of health spending on employers, businesses and citizens, and threaten to drain resources away from other policy priorities such as education, public safety and economic development.

In response, states are focusing their policy efforts on health care costs, and many of these efforts will significantly affect providers. This article summarizes key state reforms targeting medical expenses and highlights the implications for hospitals and health systems in three areas: (1) rising costs from consolidation, (2) drug price increases and (3) affordability for consumers. In the near term, the growing role of states will mean more state-by-state variation. Thus, health care organizations must focus not just on federal developments but on a proliferation of state policies that will affect their facilities, finances and delivery models.

Rising Costs from Consolidation

The latest *Futurescan* national survey of health care leaders indicates that the rapid pace of consolidation continues. Twenty-three percent of survey respondents are currently involved in a nonhorizontal merger with physicians, health plans, nonhospital facilities or health systems in different geographic areas, and nearly half of respondents are either somewhat or very likely to pursue such a combination.

As noted in prior editions of *Futurescan*, value-based payment reforms have spurred a wave of provider consolidations because the capacity to assume greater financial risk increases with a health system's scale and scope (Chernew 2017; Kaufman 2017). Nevertheless, data show that horizontal hospital mergers and vertical acquisitions of physician practices can be associated with significantly higher prices and per-patient spending as a result of market concentration, the ability to charge facility fees for acquired physicians' outpatient services and incentives to refer patients to higher-priced providers in a consolidated system (Capps, Dranove and Ody 2018; Gaynor and Town 2012; Neprash et al. 2015).

In the face of widespread health care industry consolidation, states are pursuing a variety of policy tools to address rising medical costs, including (1) policies to encourage competition

About the Author

Erin C. Fuse Brown, J.D., is an associate professor of law and a faculty member of the Center for Law, Health and Society at the Georgia State University College of Law. She has advised the National Academy for State Health Policy and the Milbank Memorial Fund on issues of state health law and policy, health care consolidation and costs. Fuse Brown has published articles in legal and medical journals on health care prices, medical billing and collection, health care competition and consolidation and consumer financial protection in health care. She is a coauthor of the eighth edition of the legal text *Health Law: Cases, Materials and Problems* (West Academic, 2018). She received a J.D. from Georgetown University Law Center, an M.P.H. from the Johns Hopkins University Bloomberg School of Public Health, and a B.A. from Dartmouth College.

FUTURESCAN SURVEY RESULTS
Policy and Regulation

How likely is it that the following will happen by 2024?

Already Happening (%)	Very Likely (%)	Somewhat Likely (%)	Neutral (%)	Somewhat Unlikely (%)	Very Unlikely (%)
23	28	21	14	7	6

Our organization will participate in a nonhorizontal merger (e.g., with physicians, a health plan, nonhospital facilities or health systems in different geographic areas).

Already Happening (%)	Very Likely (%)	Somewhat Likely (%)	Neutral (%)	Somewhat Unlikely (%)	Very Unlikely (%)
16	27	25	25	4	3

Our organization will take steps to reduce out-of-network billing of patients by 25 percent or more.

Already Happening (%)	Very Likely (%)	Somewhat Likely (%)	Neutral (%)	Somewhat Unlikely (%)	Very Unlikely (%)
18	41	28	8	5	1

Our organization will see uncompensated care costs increase by 10 percent or more.

Already Happening (%)	Very Likely (%)	Somewhat Likely (%)	Neutral (%)	Somewhat Unlikely (%)	Very Unlikely (%)
11	36	27	16	6	4

Our organization will be subject to government rate regulation or oversight that affects our commercial rates (i.e., rates offered to commercial insurance providers rather than government payers).

Already Happening (%)	Very Likely (%)	Somewhat Likely (%)	Neutral (%)	Somewhat Unlikely (%)	Very Unlikely (%)
17	35	28	13	6	1

Our organization will enter into new approaches (e.g., generic drug manufacturing or shared purchasing) or seek new suppliers of prescription drugs to address rising drug prices.

Note: Percentages in each row may not sum exactly to 100 percent because of rounding.

What Health Care Executives Anticipate by 2024

- Seventy-four percent of health care leaders believe it is at least somewhat likely their hospital or health system will be subject to government rate regulation or oversight that affects its commercial insurance rates.

- More than half (51 percent) of leaders say their organization already has participated in a nonhorizontal merger or is very likely to do so.

- Nearly nine in 10 executives (87 percent) indicate their organization is at least somewhat likely to see uncompensated care costs increase by 10 percent or more.

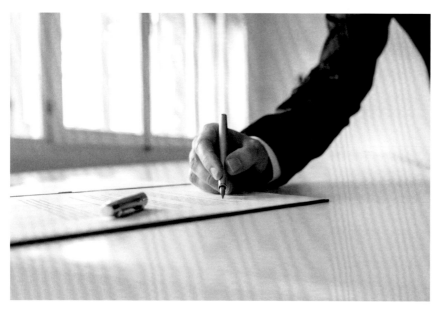

—continued from pg. 36

and market entry, (2) antitrust enforcement to block anticompetitive mergers and conduct and (3) rate regulation.

Policies to encourage competition and market entry. These policies include promoting health care price transparency, expanding scope-of-practice laws, facilitating telemedicine and reforming certificate-of-need laws. The common idea underlying all of these strategies is to encourage competition among existing providers and promote market entry by new players. However, none of these efforts changes the fact that, in most places, opening a new hospital facility is difficult because of regulatory constraints, licensing and other requirements. Thus, most health care organizations seeking to increase their scale will still turn to consolidation with other providers.

Antitrust enforcement. State attorneys general, the Federal Trade Commission and the U.S. Department of Justice have parallel enforcement authority to oppose mergers that will substantially lessen competition and to police anticompetitive conduct such as most-favored-nations clauses and price-fixing agreements. The federal antitrust enforcement agencies have been emboldened by recent successes in blocking horizontal

mergers of hospitals and health insurance companies. But fewer established theories exist to oppose vertical mergers among different services in the health care supply chain, such as hospitals' acquisition of physician groups or the megamergers involving CVS and Aetna or Express Scripts and Cigna. State attorneys general and state insurance departments may end up being more aggressive than the federal government in opposing these vertical mergers.

Rate regulation. Where hospital markets are already highly concentrated, antitrust enforcement cannot effectively restore competition, so states may seek to regulate health care rates more directly. States with concentrated markets may show growing interest in all-payer rate setting, global budgets, rate caps or site-neutral payments (Sharfstein et al. 2017). In rural areas that struggle to maintain providers, states may be interested in Certificates of Public Advantage (COPAs), which shield mergers from antitrust enforcement if the merging entities commit to keeping facilities open and investing in population health and agree to ongoing state supervision of prices and anticompetitive behavior (Greaney 2017). COPAs are a narrower form of rate regulation, offered to one health system in a merger in exchange for antitrust immunity. As

competition diminishes, state-based rate regulation may be an emerging future trend. Although only 11 percent of hospital and health system executives responding to the *Futurescan* survey report that their state currently regulates their commercial rates, 63 percent believe that state rate regulation is somewhat to very likely in the next five years.

Drug Price Increases

Rising inpatient drug prices are having a significant adverse effect on hospitals' ability to manage their costs (NORC at the University of Chicago 2016). States have been actively seeking to control the increases with some of the same policy tools used to address health care prices: transparency, antitrust enforcement and rate regulation. By the end of the 2018 legislative session, six states had passed transparency laws requiring drug manufacturers to report information underlying prescription medication price increases (National Academy for State Health Policy 2018b). Following Maryland's lead, several states are seeking additional authority for broader rate setting or to fight price gouging for extraordinary hikes (National Academy for State Health Policy 2018a). In 2018, Vermont became the first state to approve drug importation from Canada. If Vermont secures federal approval, other states will likely follow. At every turn, the pharmaceutical industry has been aggressively challenging these state drug-pricing laws in court. The ultimate breadth and reach of states' efforts to contain costs thus depends on the outcomes of pending court decisions across the country.

In addition to state regulation, hospitals are pursuing their own strategies to manage prescription drug expenses, with some systems entering the generic drug manufacturing market. Seventeen percent of executives responding to the *Futurescan* survey report they are currently seeking new approaches or new suppliers to address rising drug prices, and an additional 63 percent indicate they are somewhat or very likely to do so by 2024.

Affordability for Consumers

Affordability is emerging as the top concern of health care consumers (Jost 2016). States are responding in ways that have implications for providers. From a consumer perspective, affordability is a function of health care coverage and out-of-pocket spending. From a provider perspective, the consequence of unaffordability is a growing level of uncompensated care.

Historic coverage gains following implementation of the ACA resulted in a reduced burden of uncompensated care and improved finances for hospitals, particularly in states that expanded Medicaid (Blavin 2016; Dranove, Garthwaite and Ody 2016). But the continued proliferation of high-deductible health plans and destabilization of the individual insurance markets mean that many hospitals have again begun to experience rising levels of uncompensated care. Nearly a fifth of *Futurescan* survey respondents are already seeing their uncompensated care burden increase by 10 percent or more, and 41 percent of those surveyed believe it is very likely that uncompensated care costs will rise.

States could take the following steps to lessen the burden on providers (Jost 2018):

- Shoring up their individual insurance markets through regulation where federal supports fall away through reinsurance programs.
- Implementing a state individual mandate.
- Restricting short-term or association health plans that drain healthy people from the risk pool.

In addition, some states that have not yet expanded Medicaid will likely continue to explore ways to gain access to federal Medicaid dollars through waivers or even ballot initiatives.

States are also passing laws to protect consumers from surprise out-of-network bills. Even in the absence of state regulation, many providers are taking steps to curtail this practice. In the *Futurescan*

survey, 16 percent of respondents report taking steps to reduce out-of-network bills by 25 percent or more, while more than half say it is somewhat to very likely they will do so in the next five years. Though many surprise medical bills are generated by physicians, hospitals face significant negative publicity if their staff doctors do not participate in the same provider networks as the hospital. Further, a hospital's tax-exempt status may be threatened if its contracted emergency department (ED) physicians do not follow the hospital's financial assistance policy and engage in aggressive patient billing and collection practices.

Hospital and health system leaders should be mindful of the likely role of states in setting health policy and regulating the health care industry.

Implications for Health Care Leaders

For the near term, hospital and health system leaders should be mindful of the following trends regarding the likely role of states in setting health policy and regulating the health care industry.

States are targeting health care consolidation. Providers should expect state antitrust enforcement authorities and insurance regulators to oppose the potentially harmful competitive effects of some health care mergers and megamergers. Antitrust enforcers may also begin to police vertical mergers involving health care organizations, such as hospital–physician practice acquisitions or hospital–health plan mergers. In rural areas, states may be willing to protect merging providers with COPAs to promote health care integration and population health and to prevent hospital closures. These mergers are usually provider driven but come with long-term state oversight and

regulation. Where consolidation has already occurred and competition can no longer keep rising prices in check, states may use rate regulation tools such as all-payer models or global hospital budgets.

States are at the forefront of efforts to control drug pricing, and pharmaceutical manufacturers are fighting back. States are actively pursuing legislation to combat the rising cost of prescription medications, including laws to increase transparency about manufacturers' and pharmacy benefit managers' expenses, anti-price-gouging laws, drug price regulation and importation of prescription

drugs from Canada. States are facing a well-funded counterattack in the courts by the pharmaceutical industry. Hospitals can collaborate with their state legislatures to maximize the effectiveness of initiatives that seek to limit increases in inpatient drug prices and to fight efforts by pharmaceutical trade groups to stop them.

Providers should be concerned about consumer health care affordability. States are taking action to improve consumer affordability's twin drivers: health care coverage and out-of-pocket spending. Health care coverage is as critical to providers' fiscal health as it is to the health of the communities they serve. Studies show that Medicaid expansion—which is being considered by a growing number of states—strengthens hospital finances, protects rural providers from closure and reduces uncompensated care. Similar positive results are likely in states that take steps to protect their individual insurance markets from destabilization caused by federal administration policies. In addition, more states are cracking down on surprise medical billing. Hospitals can take action to address the issue by working with staff doctors and contracted ED physicians to reduce or eliminate the controversial practice.

Conclusion

States are actively seeking ways to address rising medical costs on many fronts. Hospital and health system leaders who proactively strive to minimize the impact of health care costs on consumers and communities will be better able to partner with their state policymakers in crafting solutions.

References

Blavin, F. 2016. "Association Between the 2014 Medicaid Expansion and U.S. Hospital Finances." *Journal of the American Medical Association* 316 (14): 1475–83.

Capps, C., D. Dranove and C. Ody. 2018. "The Effect of Hospital Acquisitions of Physician Practices on Prices and Spending." *Journal of Health Economics* 59: 139–52.

Chernew, M. 2017. "Two Payment Models Will Dominate the Move to Value-Based Care." In *Futurescan 2017–2022: Healthcare Trends and Implications*, 12–16. Chicago: Society for Healthcare Strategy & Market Development of the American Hospital Association and the American College of Healthcare Executives.

Dranove, D., C. Garthwaite and C. Ody. 2016. "Uncompensated Care Decreased at Hospitals in Medicaid Expansion States but Not at Hospitals in Nonexpansion States." *Health Affairs* 35 (8): 1471–79.

Gaynor, M., and R. Town. 2012. *The Impact of Hospital Consolidation—Update*. Robert Wood Johnson Foundation. Published June. www.rwjf.org/content/dam/farm/reports/issue_briefs/2012/rwjf73261.

Greaney, T.L. 2017. "Coping with Concentration." *Health Affairs* 36 (9): 1564–71.

Jost, T.S. 2018. "Market Stabilization Stalls; States Step In." *Health Affairs* 37 (6): 848–49.

———. 2016. "Affordability: The Most Urgent Health Reform Issue for Ordinary Americans." *Health Affairs Blog*. Published February 29. www.healthaffairs.org/do/10.1377/hblog20160229.053330/full/.

Kaufman, K. 2017. "The New Role of Healthcare Integration." In *Futurescan 2017–2022: Healthcare Trends and Implications*, 7–11. Chicago: Society for Healthcare Strategy & Market Development of the American Hospital Association and the American College of Healthcare Executives.

National Academy for State Health Policy. 2018a. "States' Prescription Drug Transparency Laws Open the Black Box of Drug Pricing." Published June. https://nashp.org/state-rx-price-transparency-laws-open-the-black-box-of-drug-pricing/.

———. 2018b. "While the Administration Mulls How to Curb Prescription Costs, State Legislatures Take the Lead." Published May. https://nashp.org/while-the-administration-mulls-how-to-curb-drug-costs-state-legislatures-are-acting/.

Neprash, H.T., M.E. Chernew, A.L. Hicks, T. Gibson and J.M. McWilliams. 2015. "Association of Financial Integration Between Physicians and Hospitals with Commercial Health Care Prices." *JAMA Internal Medicine* 175 (12): 1932–39.

NORC at the University of Chicago. 2016. *Trends in Hospital Inpatient Drug Costs: Issues and Challenges*. Presented to the American Hospital Association. Published October 11. www.aha.org/system/files/2018-01/aha-fah-rx-report.pdf.

Sharfstein, J., S. Gerovich, E. Moriarty and D. Chin. 2017. *An Emerging Approach to Payment Reform: All-Payer Global Budgets for Large Safety-Net Hospital Systems*. The Commonwealth Fund. Published August. www.commonwealthfund.org/publications/fund-reports/2017/aug/emerging-approach-payment-reform-all-payer-global-budgets-large.

Solutions to Workforce Shortages May Require Strategic Partners

by Susan Salka

Workforce challenges—most notably unprecedented shortages of qualified staff—pose a critical issue for health care organizations today and in the future. Leaders are acutely aware of these challenges, particularly given that employees have the most direct impact on patient outcomes and represent more than half of their operating budget, and thus their single largest expense (Fitch Ratings 2016). Yet, many hospitals and health systems are ill prepared to deal with the shortages, which are occurring among all types of health care professionals in almost all regions of the country and are driving problems related to hiring, retention, turnover, unit staffing and scheduling, morale, quality of care and overtime costs.

One reason is that the majority of hospital human resources departments are underfunded; expenditures usually tally only 1 percent of operating budgets (Bloomberg BNA 2015), with spending on talent acquisition and retention being only a fraction of that amount. Consequently, the considerable investment required for technology-enabled

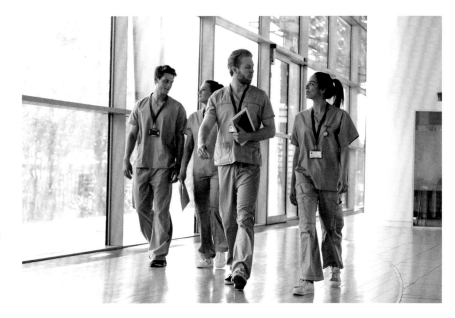

solutions and development of advanced staffing expertise may be beyond the operational capabilities of most health care organizations. Today's potential clinical candidates, most of whom already have jobs, must be engaged through very contemporary ways, including via multiple (and costly) digital platforms and internet channels. Addressing 21st century health care

workforce issues thus requires considerable expenses outside of patient care.

Evidence of Persistent Shortages

As CEO and president of AMN Healthcare, a provider of health care staffing services, I see firsthand the worsening struggles health care organizations are facing to find and keep the staff they

About the Author

Susan Salka is president and CEO of AMN Healthcare Services Inc. Under her leadership, AMN has become an innovator in health care workforce solutions and the largest and most diversified health care staffing company in the nation. She is passionate about and actively involved in corporate social responsibility, diversity and inclusion, and gender equality. She personally participates in many of the company's community initiatives, including its annual medical and community development mission trip to the impoverished regions of Guatemala. A

member of Women Business Leaders and the Women Corporate Directors Foundation, Salka is a proponent of promoting women in leadership. She has made gender equality a priority since joining AMN, and in 2018 the company was named to the Bloomberg Gender-Equality Index and the Human Rights Campaign Foundation's Corporate Equality Index. She currently serves on the board of directors of McKesson, a Fortune #5 company. An alumna of Chadron State College, she received her master's degree in finance from San Diego State University.

Workforce

How likely is it that the following will happen by 2024?

Already Happening (%)	Very Likely (%)	Somewhat Likely (%)	Neutral (%)	Somewhat Unlikely (%)	Very Unlikely (%)		
43		34		15	3	4	0

Workforce shortages will be one of the three most significant challenges facing our organization.

39		33		18	3	4	3

Our organization will increase employment of advanced practice clinicians (also known as physician extenders) by at least 20 percent.

39		27		22	6	4	1

Our organization will take steps (e.g., increasing staff engagement, raising salaries or expanding our recruitment budget) to compete for staff with emerging ambulatory care providers such as home health care and retail care (e.g., retail clinics).

9	31	23	14	14	8

Our human resources department will use advanced data analysis tools, such as artificial intelligence or predictive analytics, to identify opportunities or potential actions to reduce turnover of clinical staff.

16	26	24	16	13	4

Our organization will increasingly partner with external health care staffing experts to ensure the optimization of our workforce.

Note: Percentages in each row may not sum exactly to 100 percent because of rounding.

What Health Care Executives Anticipate by 2024

- Most health care executives (77 percent) indicate workforce shortages either already are or are very likely to be one of the three most significant challenges facing their organization.

- Nearly nine in 10 respondents (88 percent) are at least somewhat likely to implement strategies such as increasing staff engagement, raising salaries or expanding their recruitment budget to compete with emerging health care providers in the race to acquire talent.

- Two-thirds of hospital and health system leaders either already are partnering with outside staffing experts to optimize their workforce or are at least somewhat likely to do so.

—continued from pg. 41

need. Evidence strongly suggests that the shortages will persist, or even worsen, in the foreseeable future. U.S. Bureau of Labor Statistics (BLS) data show that demand for all practitioners and technical occupations in health care will remain strong for the next decade even as job openings continue to grow, resulting in a cumulative glut of unfilled positions facing healthcare organizations.

Health care employment growth. According to the BLS, health care employment growth has been on a steady upward trajectory for the past decade, increasing from 13.3 million jobs in 2008 to 16 million in 2018 (exhibit 1). With the exception of two months in 2013 and one month in 2014, employment growth has continued even through the worst economic recession since the Great Depression (BLS 2018a). Such momentum over a long period of time is a clear sign of robust and enduring demand for health care professionals.

Growing gap of unfilled jobs. Another strong indicator of high demand comes from the BLS's Job Openings and Labor Turnover Survey. Although openings have traditionally outpaced hires in health care, the gap has been rapidly widening since 2014, with monthly openings rising and hires remaining relatively static (exhibit 2).

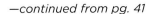

Exhibit 1

Health Care Employment Growth

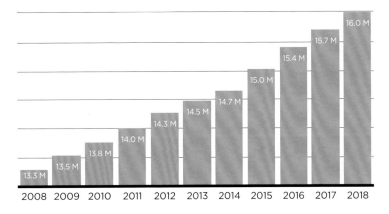

Source: BLS (2018b).

Exhibit 2

Growing Gap Between Job Openings and Job Hires in Health Care

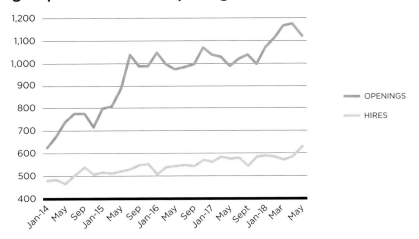

Source: BLS (2018d).
Note: In thousands.

Expected job openings per year. Projected job openings—which includes new positions as well as retirements, resignations and other types of job separation—may be the most important data point for gauging demand for health care services and workers. These are the jobs that providers will make it a priority to fill in the future. The BLS's 2016–2026 employment survey forecasts a startling 1.26 million total health care job openings per year (exhibit 3). For all practitioners and technical occupations, there will be 624,000 vacancies per year, including 204,000 openings for registered nurses (RNs) (BLS 2017). Such sizeable numbers of future job openings clearly show strong and sustained demand.

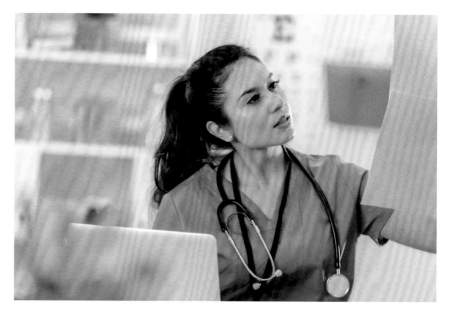

Leading Drivers of Escalating Demand

The greatest driver of increased long-range demand for health care services and workers is the aging of America. According to projections from the U.S. Census Bureau, the number of people aged 65 or older will grow from 43 million in 2012 to 84 million in 2050—that is, from 14 percent of the population to 21 percent (Ortman, Velkoff and Hogan 2014). And because the elderly require both a greater quantity and a greater complexity of care and are more likely to use skilled nursing, medical expenses for this age group are approximately three times higher than those for the average working-age adult, and about five times higher than those for the average child (Lassman et al. 2014).

Another factor fueling the trend is the wave of retirements among baby boomers. Evidence from an AMN Healthcare survey of RNs suggests this wave has already begun (AMN Healthcare 2017). From 2015 to 2017, the percentage of RNs who planned to retire in less than a year nearly doubled. Retirements are also expected to take a toll on the future supply of physicians, as more than a third of today's practicing doctors will turn 65 within the next 10 years (Mann 2017).

Exhibit 3

Average Annual Job Openings, 2016–2026

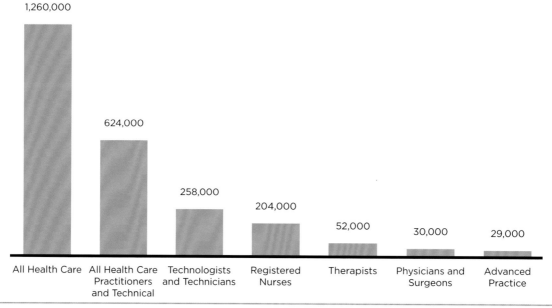

Source: BLS (2017).

Shortage Projections

Based on these factors, the health care field is projected to experience the following severe shortages in the near future:

- The American Association of Medical Colleges estimates a possible shortage of more than 100,000 physicians by 2030 (Mann 2017).
- Various research reports forecast significant nursing shortages, including a deficit of more than 150,000 RNs by 2020 and more than 500,000 by 2030 (Zhang et al. 2018). Another report predicts a shortfall of 193,000 nurses by 2020 (Carnevale, Smith and Gulish 2015).
- Because of budget constraints and a lack of faculty, clinical sites, classroom space and clinical preceptors, U.S. nursing schools turned away 64,067 qualified applicants in 2016 and 2017 (Fang et al. 2017).
- Supply-and-demand models predict a shortage of 26,560 physical therapists by 2025 (American Physical Therapy Association 2017).
- By 2025, the nation will likely face a shortage of 29,400 nurse practitioners and 98,700 medical and lab technologists and technicians (Stevenson 2018).

Insights from the *Futurescan* Survey

The latest *Futurescan* survey indicates that health care executives' opinions about potential solutions to the staffing shortage vary considerably.

Most respondents (66 percent) reported that their organization is already budgeting or is very likely to budget more money for traditional, internal solutions to compete with emerging ambulatory care providers for talent, such as raising salaries and spending more on recruitment and staff engagement. These strategies, however, do not increase the total available pool of clinical candidates for health care organizations. Recruiting by one organization may create a staffing gap at another institution.

A significantly smaller number of respondents (9 percent) said they are already using advanced, technology-enabled solutions, such as artificial intelligence and predictive analytics, to reduce turnover of clinical staff. However, another 31 percent predict they are very likely to do so in the next five years.

Sixteen percent are partnering with external health care staffing experts to optimize their workforce, while 26 percent said they are very likely to do so by 2024.

Implications for Health Care Leaders

The workforce crisis will be a fact of life in health care for the foreseeable future. This formidable challenge for providers comes on top of other difficulties, including shifting regulatory and reimbursement policies that strain an organization's revenue cycle and ability to deliver value-based care.

As a result, I believe many hospital and health system executives may balk at focusing exclusively on internal

Successful Organizations Are Using a Combination of Strategies to Address Health Care Workforce Shortages

by Denise J. Mariotti

Solving workforce shortages is a top priority for executives in the rapidly changing health care environment. In fact, the vast majority of those responding to the latest *Futurescan* survey indicate it is or is very likely to be one of their three most significant challenges over the next five years.

The problem calls for leaders to both maximize existing approaches and embrace new ways of acquiring top talent. To remain competitive, health care organizations must use innovative strategies for talent acquisition and retention, including the following:

- Increasing the strategic workforce-planning management skills of human resources professionals.
- Offering competitive compensation for in-demand health care positions and medical professionals (e.g., nurses, employed physicians).
- Strengthening recruitment efforts.
  - Using modern communication channels (e.g., social media).
  - Attracting and meeting the needs of employees of different age generations, including Gen Z, Gen Y (millennials) and Gen X.
  - Creating opportunities for veterans with health care experience.
- Investing in retention by improving the new-employee onboarding process and increasing staff engagement and professional development opportunities.
- Educating students at an early age about the broad range of careers available in health care.
- Partnering with local colleges and universities to establish educational programs for nursing and other health care professions that can serve as hiring pipelines.
- Offering paid internships, fellowships, mentoring programs, job shadowing, tuition assistance/reimbursement and loan forgiveness.

(continued)

tactics or implementing technology-driven approaches on their own. In fact, record averages of weekly hours worked and high workforce attrition rates point to an increase in the use of overtime for clinical staff (BLS 2018c). These red flags suggest that health care organizations are increasingly turning to stopgap measures to deal with workforce supply problems.

> The American Association of Medical Colleges estimates a possible shortage of more than 100,000 physicians by 2030.

Best practices in attracting high-quality clinical staff have changed dramatically in recent years. Relying on a Rolodex, telephone directory, job boards, job fairs and personal contacts does not work today. Health care recruitment and hiring in the information age require new approaches:

- Establishing a national strategy and operation for digital workforce sourcing.
- Utilizing hundreds of social media channels, search engines and websites.
- Engaging with candidates and employees through digital and mobile platforms.
- Tapping into the largest available database of health care professionals.
- Acquiring advanced data analytics expertise for workforce sourcing.
- Using predictive analytics to forecast patient volume months in advance.
- Implementing automation for many aspects of clinical employment.
- Using comprehensive workforce management of all supplemental staff.

Conclusion

Implementing these approaches can be challenging for providers as they transition to value-based care and adjust to changing regulatory and reimbursement policies. To be successful in acquiring talent during the worsening workforce shortage, many are turning to outside companies that have specialized expertise in these advancements. In my opinion, this may be the most practical and impactful solution.

(continued from previous page)

- Using new data/technology tools, such as predictive analytics.
- Increasing the hiring of advanced practice clinicians, such as physician assistants and nurse practitioners.
- Helping physicians, nurses and other employees find "joy in practice" and reduce job burnout.
- Developing clinical education and training programs that are unique and accessible.
- Identifying opportunities for employees nearing retirement age to continue to work full- or part-time.
- Redesigning work processes to increase efficiency and employee satisfaction.
- Leveraging the expertise of outside experts who specialize in workforce solutions.

The looming crisis requires human resources professionals and clinical and nonclinical executives who are willing to lead change, adopt creative best practices, build a culture of employee engagement and adapt their management style to the new generations of workers.

Today, there is no one right way or formula for health care organizations to address workforce shortages. Forward-thinking hospitals and health systems are making strides in acquiring and retaining talent by using a combination of internal and external initiatives that are right for their particular staffing needs in their unique market.

Ultimately, the effectiveness of workforce strategies will be driven by leaders who recognize that these approaches can have a positive impact on solving the shortages, and who empower and engage employees at all levels of the organization to provide the best patient care.

About the Author

Denise J. Mariotti is the chief human resources officer at the Hospital of the University of Pennsylvania. She has worked in a variety of human resources leadership roles at Penn Medicine for nearly 20 years. She received a bachelor of arts degree from Rosemont College. Mariotti has been awarded numerous certificates and honors, including the Pennsylvania Governor's Achievement Award for Outstanding Performance in Job Training and Placement.

References

American Physical Therapy Association. 2017. "A Model to Project the Supply and Demand of Physical Therapists: 2010–2025." Updated April 17. www.apta.org/WorkforceData/ModelDescriptionFigures/.

AMN Healthcare. 2017. *2017 Survey of Registered Nurses: Viewpoints on Leadership, Nursing Shortages, and Their Profession*. San Diego, CA: AMN Healthcare.

Bloomberg BNA. 2015. *HR Department Benchmarks and Analysis, 2015–2016*. Accessed July 24, 2018. www.bna.com/uploadedFiles/BNA_V2/HR/Products/Surveys_and_Reports/HR%20Department%20Benchmark%20and%20Analysis%202015-16_Executive%20Summary.pdf.

Carnevale, A., N. Smith and A. Gulish. 2015. "Nursing Supply and Demand Through 2020." Georgetown University Center on Education and the Workforce. Accessed July 24, 2018. https://cew.georgetown.edu/cew-reports/nursingprojections/.

Fang, D., Y. Li, K.A. Kennedy and D.E. Trautman. 2017. *2016–2017 Enrollment and Graduations in Baccalaureate and Graduate Programs in Nursing*. Washington, DC: American Association of Colleges of Nursing.

Fitch Ratings. 2016. *2016 Median Ratios for Nonprofit Hospitals and Healthcare Systems: Special Report*. Published September 9. www.fitchratings.com/site/re/887525.

Lassman, D., M. Hartman, B. Washington, K. Andrews and A. Catlin. 2014. "US Health Spending Trends by Age and Gender: Selected Years 2002–10." *Health Affairs* 33 (5): 815–22.

Mann, S. 2017. "Research Shows Shortage of More Than 100,000 Doctors by 2030." *AAMC News*. Published March 14. https://news.aamc.org/medical-education/article/new-aamc-research-reaffirms-looming-physician-shor/.

Ortman, J.M., V.A. Velkoff and H. Hogan. 2014. "An Aging Nation: The Older Population in the United States." Published May. www.census.gov/prod/2014pubs/p25-1140.pdf.

Stevenson, M. 2018. *Demand for Healthcare Workers Will Outpace Supply by 2025: An Analysis of the US Healthcare Labor Market*. Mercer LLC. Accessed November 15. www.mercer.com/content/dam/mercer/attachments/private/gl-career-2018-demand-for-healthcare-workers-will-outpace-supply-by-2025-analyisis-healthcare-labor-market-mercer.pdf.

US Bureau of Labor Statistics. 2018a. "Employment, Hours, and Earnings from the Current Employment Statistics Survey (National). 1-Month Net Change. All Employees, Health Care, Seasonally Adjusted." Current Employment Statistics (CES) multiscreen data search. Data extracted November 17. www.bls.gov/ces/.

———. 2018b. "Employment, Hours, and Earnings from the Current Employment Statistics Survey (National). All Employees, Health Care, Seasonally Adjusted." Current Employment Statistics (CES) multiscreen data search. Data extracted November 27. www.bls.gov/ces/.

———. 2018c. "Employment, Hours, and Earnings from the Current Employment Statistics Survey (National). Average Weekly Hours of All Employees, Health Care, Seasonally Adjusted." Current Employment Statistics (CES) multiscreen data search. Data extracted November 27. www.bls.gov/ces/.

———. 2018d. "Hires, Job Openings, Health Care and Social Assistance, Seasonally Adjusted." Job Openings and Labor Turnover Survey (JOLTS) multiscreen data search. Data extracted November 27. www.bls.gov/jlt/.

———. 2017. "Employment Projections: Employment by Detailed Occupation, 2016 and Projected 2026." Data extracted July 10, 2018. www.bls.gov/emp/tables/emp-by-detailed-occupation.htm.

Zhang, X., D. Tai, H. Pforsich and V.W. Lin. 2018. "United States Registered Nurse Workforce Report Card and Shortage Forecast: A Revisit." *American Journal of Medical Quality* 33 (3): 229–36.

Society for Healthcare Strategy & Market Development

    Executive director: Diane Weber, RN
    Managing editor: Brian Griffin
    Research data analytics specialist: Ann Feeney

The Society for Health Care Strategy & Market Development (SHSMD) of the American Hospital Association is the largest and most prominent voice for health care strategists in marketing, planning, business development, communications, public relations and physician strategy.

SHSMD is committed to leading, connecting, and serving its members to prepare them for the future with greater knowledge and opportunity as their organizations strive to improve the health of their communities. The society provides a broad and constantly updated array of resources, services, experiences and connections.

SHSMD leaders are available for on-site presentations about *Futurescan 2019–2024* to health care governing boards, senior management, planning teams and medical staffs. To arrange for a leadership presentation, contact SHSMD at 312.422.3888 or shsmd@aha.org.

American College of Healthcare Executives/Health Administration Press

    President and CEO: Deborah J. Bowen, FACHE, CAE
    Director, Health Administration Press: Michael E. Cunningham, CAE
    Project manager: Andrew J. Baumann
    Layout editor: Cepheus Edmondson

The American College of Healthcare Executives is an international professional society of more than 48,000 healthcare executives who lead hospitals, healthcare systems and other healthcare organizations. ACHE's mission is to advance its members and healthcare management excellence. ACHE offers its prestigious FACHE® credential, signifying board certification in healthcare management. ACHE's established network of 78 chapters provides access to networking, education and career development at the local level. In addition, ACHE is known for its magazine, *Healthcare Executive*, and its career development and public policy programs. Through such efforts, ACHE works toward its vision of being the preeminent professional society for leaders dedicated to improving health.

The Foundation of the American College of Healthcare Executives was established to further advance healthcare management excellence through education and research. The Foundation of ACHE is known for its educational programs—including the annual Congress on Healthcare Leadership, which draws more than 4,000 participants—and groundbreaking research. Its publishing division, Health Administration Press, is one of the largest publishers of books and journals on health services management, including textbooks for college and university courses. For more information, visit www.ache.org.

CareTech Solutions is a leader in information technology (IT) and end-user interface services for more than 200 hospitals and health systems across the country. Since 1998, its 1,400 dedicated U.S.-based experts have created value for clients through customized IT solutions that contribute to improving the patient experience while lowering health care costs. CareTech Solutions is a health IT subsidiary of HTC Global, a global provider of IT solutions and business process outsourcing services. For more information, visit www.caretech.com.